the modern
HERB GARDENER

the modern
HERB GARDENER

SALLY ROTH

CONSULTANT ROSEMARY TITTERINGTON

CARROLL & BROWN PUBLISHERS LIMITED

First published in 2001 in the United Kingdom by:

Carroll & Brown Publishers Limited
20 Lonsdale Road
Queen's Park
London NW6 6RD

Editor Charlotte Beech
Managing Art Editor Adelle Morris
Design Assistant Roland Codd

Illustrations and compilation © 2001 Carroll & Brown Limited
Text © 2001 Sally Roth

A CIP catalogue record for this book is available from the British Library.

ISBN 1-903258-22-7

Reproduced by Emirates in Dubai
Printed and bound by Imago in Singapore

First edition

This is not a medical reference book. The information it contains is general, not specific to
individuals. Any plant substance, whether used as food or medicine, externally or internally,
can cause an allergic reaction in some people. Neither the author nor the publishers shall be
held liable or responsible for any claims arising from the mistaken identity of any herbs, or
the inappropriate use of any remedy.

Contents

why herbs?

As beautiful as any plants in the garden, herbs are steeped in centuries of history and romance. A plant's usefulness is what classifies it as a herb, whether it's a sprig of thyme simmered in a stew or a few stems of lavender laid between the sheets. The uses for herbs are almost as endless as the variety of these plants. Every culture has its favourites, which it uses to flavour food and drink, heal a multitude of human ailments, make the home smell better, discourage pests and even improve personal appearance or smooth the skin.

Knowing the stories behind herbs and using them in everyday activities makes these plants a very personal part of your garden. But usefulness is only part of the reason herbs are favourites in gardens. These plants are also beautiful, with delightfully fragrant leaves and often delicate flowers. Because many popular herbs have lovely foliage in soft greys and greens and understated flowers, you'll find that combining them is simple: everything looks good together, so designing an attractive garden is easy. You can slip herbs in amongst ornamentals, or keep them handy in a special patch of, say, culinary herbs or a tea garden. Growing herbs can also give you a healthier garden, thanks to their pest-repelling ability. What's more, their blossoms attract beneficial insects, which will patrol other parts of your garden to destroy harmful insects.

So many plants have been used as herbs around the globe that, chances are, your garden already includes a plentiful sampling of them. Those dandelions that dot the green grass of spring, for instance, were regulars in the medicine chests of long-ago herbal practitioners, who valued them for their cure-almost-all properties. The flamboyant rose bushes that pretty up your ornamental beds in summer can similarly be called herbs, because they were once used in order to ward off colds and flu.

Use this book to help you decide which herbs to choose, where to plant them and how to care for them so they enjoy a long and useful life. Browse through the directory in chapter 5 to discover old favourites and intriguing new herbs to try in your own garden. You'll learn how to harvest and store your herbs, too, so that you can enjoy using them in the many recipes and project ideas you'll come across in these pages. One word of caution: gardening with herbs is so much fun, it can quickly turn you into a dedicated collector. Experiment with just a few of these fascinating plants, and you will open the door to a gardening hobby that will last a lifetime.

Herbs are full of surprises to add a little zest to your life – a simple summer dessert can become an unusual and unexpected delight in a decorative ice bowl, complete with edible chive flowers, cucumber and mint encased in its walls

planning your garden

Starting a herb garden is often as casual as bringing home that first small pot of lavender. Soon there's a plant of rosemary nearby and an edging of creeping thyme sneaking out along the stepping stones. That's a fine beginning, but for the most satisfying garden, it helps to do a bit of daydreaming before you pick up the trowel and load up the car boot.

a home for herbs

No matter how small or how grand your garden, there's a place for herbs – which is a good thing, because herb gardens have a habit of expanding as you come across exciting new plants to try. Read on to discover how to make the most of your garden space.

Herbs thrive in all kinds of settings. They flourish in containers as well as planted in the garden, can snuggle into niches between stepping stones or fill entire beds. Start by thinking about how you plan to use your herbs. If cooking is high on the list, you'll want the culinary herbs near the kitchen door so you can snip a few stems of parsley or chives without making a major expedition. If you're planning to decorate your home with herbs in dried arrangements or potpourri, you'll want those herbs where you can easily reach them, perhaps in a special cutting garden or at least near a path.

Notice which gardens in this book appeal to you most. Is your eye attracted to the cottage-style jumble, the simplicity of plants in classic pots or the intricate curves of a knot garden? Many herb gardeners like to keep their collection in a separate herbs-only garden, a place that quickly becomes a gathering of old and new plant friends. Others choose to mingle herbs and flowers, planting parsley or thyme as an edging to ornamentals. Most of us mix it up, keeping some favourite herbs in their own space and moving others to any suitable spot. You'll find an abundance of ideas in the following pages to help you decide what kinds of gardens suit your style.

Practical considerations are vital too. Herbs originally hail from regions all around the world, so you'll find many plants that will thrive in your garden, whatever your climate. Select those that suit your region and your growing conditions, just as you would any other garden plant. Sun and well-drained soil are the basics for many herbs, but others will thrive in shade, heavy clay or even particularly wet soils.

basil

bay

cardamom

chives

dill

lemon verbena

parsley

rosemary

sage

thyme

indoors

A sunny windowsill gives you enough growing room to keep a fine collection of cooking herbs for the kitchen: parsley, sage, rosemary and thyme, perhaps oregano for livening up the pizza and chives for Sunday-morning scrambled eggs. It's a cook's dream in just half a metre of shelf space. Basil is an easy candidate for windowsill culture because the seeds sprout fast and the plants grow to usable size in a matter of weeks.

There is no need to stop with the kitchen, either. Use lavender or scented geraniums as a natural air freshener for your living room, or in the bath, where you can add a few leaves to steaming water for a fragrant, relaxing soak.

If you live in a cold-winter area, move tender potted herbs indoors to enjoy as houseplants on a sunny, glassed-in porch or under full-spectrum grow lights. Narrow, plastic windowbox liners fit on many indoor sills, making it a simple matter to grow annual herbs, like bright-flowered, peppery-tasting nasturtiums or feathery dill from seed.

TIPS FOR SUCCESSFUL INDOOR HERB GARDENING

- Give plants as much light as possible – south-facing windows or artificial grow lights are ideal.
- Buy young potted plants for best success. Plants moved in from the garden may have difficulty adjusting; transplant any divisions or cuttings to pots during the summer and leave them for a few weeks before the indoor move.
- Keep herbs away from heat sources.
- Pinch off the growing tips to keep the plants bushy and compact.
- Use lightweight plastic pots, so you can easily move them for cleaning or to catch more light.
- Protect floors and windowsills by placing waterproof trays underneath pots.

If you're lucky enough to have a heated sun-room or a wall consisting of mostly windows, the increased warmth and light will expand your options. Grow lemongrass or lemon verbena for teas, or try a tumble of German chamomile with its delicate, white daisies. For a specimen plant, try pineapple sage, whose pretty flowers and leaves add colour and flavour to iced beverages. Greenhouses will also protect plants in winter.

herbs in containers

Growing your plants in containers is a convenient and satisfying way to get started with outdoor herb gardening and also adds visual excitement to any garden. For a small investment in a container, potting mix and plants, you can have a handy windowbox, beautiful hanging basket or a garden centrepiece in place within an hour.

POTS

Potted plants are attention-grabbers in the garden, acting as focal points that draw the eye. To make the pot stand out even further, you could

10 best herbs for pots

basil   bay   lavender   lemongrass   lemon verbena   pansies   rosemary   sage   scented geraniums   thyme

10 best herbs for windowboxes

aloe vera

box

chamomile

lavenders

lemon verbena

marjoram

pansies

sage

scented
geraniums

thymes

set it on a wall, post or doorstep, or give it a gentle boost by perching it on top of bricks or an overturned pot. Use large pots to flank a gateway or doorstep or elevate a big pot amongst the exuberant herbs of an informal garden to help create a sense of control.

Light, fast-draining potting soil is ideal for the roots of many herbs, including popular lavender, oregano, thyme and scented geraniums. Add a few scoops of compost or some granulated water-holding polymer gel beads to reduce your watering tasks. A water-soluble balanced fertilizer or organic supplement, such as miracle grow, applied every two weeks, will keep your potted herbs flourishing in spring and early summer.

You can combine herbs of similar cultural needs, plant a sampler of different kinds of the same herb (various lavenders or thymes, for instance) or use just one herb. Fill the container with potting mix, then play with your plants until you like the arrangement. Slip them out of their pots one at a time, scoop out a hole for the root ball and gently firm them in. Leave 5 cm above the soil line to help prevent water overflowing.

WINDOWBOXES

Irresistibly charming, windowboxes are an appealing addition to your home because they bring the garden right up to your walls. The conditions are demanding, though, so you'll need to choose herbs that can survive in a difficult site. On the sunny side of your house, windowboxes

can create almost desert conditions for your herbs. The roots have little insulating soil to protect them from the full force of the sun, and the plants get extra heat reflected from the nearby glass and wall. Plastic liners are a clever way to keep windowboxes looking good. You can slip them out in seconds to give tired plants a rest and slide in a fresh replacement.

Plan to water a windowbox at least once a day in summer, preferably in the morning so that roots have enough moisture to draw on during the heat of high noon. Water-holding polymer gel beads added to the soil at planting time, or self-watering windowboxes can make life easier for your plants, and you, by providing a backup source of water when you can't get to the hose.

HANGING BASKETS

Fill hanging baskets with mounding or upright plants in the centre to balance the pot visually, and finish the arrangement with cascading herbs around the edge to make it look graceful. As in other plantings, you can stick to herbs alone or blend other plants into the design. A lacy collar of German chamomile, for example, adds a dainty contrast to the large flowers of petunias, and also looks beautiful with the scalloped grey foliage of apple-scented geranium. Houseleek makes an intriguing basket when you stud it around the sides and bottom of an open-frame container lined with spaghnum moss and filled with potting mix. They will soon cover every inch of empty space with clusters of highly textured rosettes.

Read catalogues and plant labels carefully to find good herb varieties for your hanging baskets. Depending on the cultivar, herbs such as rosemary and thyme may be upright in growth habit or they may sprawl and spread – these are the attributes you want for your basket.

Plant and care for hanging baskets as you would herbs in pots, watering them frequently and fertilizing about once a week.

TOPIARY

A neatly trimmed cone or ball of greenery is the perfect finishing touch for a formal or semi-formal garden, as the h... of the gardener is very much in control. Known as topiary, these decoratively pruned plants also make striking table centrepieces. Any herb with a single main stem and a branching habit of growth may be trained.

You can buy topiary-grown herbs in nurseries and garden centres, or you can make your own. Start with a young herb, the bushiest you can find. Prune it into the basic ...ape you want, then wait a few weeks to let new branches form. Pinch or snip off the first set of leaves from each tip to encourage more branching. Once the plant has dense new foliage, fine-tune it by selectively snipping off tender branch tips. Water as ...rmal but be generous with nitrogen-boosting fertilizer.

As the plant grows, maintain the shape by snipping off any wayward shoots as they appear

herbs in gardens

Spend a few minutes considering the general garden design principles of contrasting or complementing texture, shape and colour and you can use a palette of herbs to paint a garden portrait as beautiful as any ornamental planting. Foliage is an outstanding attribute of many herbs, often with deliciously soft or fine texture and a gentle range of greys and greens. Intersperse bold-leaved herbs, such as chicory or sweet Joe Pye, among daintier garden neighbours for a textural contrast that makes both partners more pleasing to the eye. Slip in an upright citizen, such as angelica or mullein, for a vertical exclamation point among more relaxed company.

ALONE AND AS PARTNERS

An all-herb garden is always satisfying because the plants share a common bond that ties them together: they're all useful for one thing or another. Many enthusiasts find pleasure in a herb garden arranged by type of use rather than ornamental design: all cooking herbs, for instance, or all curative herbs.

Adding herbs to ornamental plantings broadens their contribution to the garden. The dramatic deep red foliage of fennel or perilla, for example, adds a valuable deep note to a bed of pastel flowers. Lots of favourite garden flowers are really herbs at heart: roses, for example have many practical uses beyond looking beautiful. Throughout this book, you'll find photos and suggestions to inspire new ways to mix and mingle your herbs and flowers, whether you grow them alone or to add flair to flowerbeds.

informal gardens

A relaxed attitude comes naturally to herbs, many of which will spread, sprawl or creep instead of staying in tidy clumps. They're well suited to the casual style of informal gardens, therefore, where the lines of borders are more loose and curving, and the plants can easily blend into each other.

BORDERS

Plant herbs in borders according to their height and habit, whether you're planning a herbs-only garden or you want to mix them in with your favourite ornamentals. Tall, stout herbs with large leaves, such as angelica and Joe Pye weed, are best positioned towards the back of borders, where they won't block the sun or your view of the shorter plants. Some tall herbs, especially annuals such as dill and caraway, have small leaves and an open habit, making them easy to see through. Plant these in the middle or even in the front of a bed or border, where their lightweight texture won't get lost in the crowd. Herbs of mounded habit, for example sage or thyme,

the kitchen garden

Keep your most-used culinary herbs close at hand by growing them in pots or a raised bed close to your kitchen door. Start with the basics – parsley, chives, dill, thyme and anything else you and your family like. Experiment with strong herbs, too, perhaps French tarragon for Friday fish dinners or coriander to jazz up a salsa. When the possibilities are right in arm's reach, you'll be much more inclined to liven up the menu. Be sure to label each plant so friends and family members can help with the harvesting.

should go in the middle, while creepers and low growers, such as chamomile or creeping thyme, look best edging the bed.

It's hard to make mistakes when combining herbs, but do try to avoid inviting aggressive spreaders, such as mint, tansy and goldenrod, into your beds and borders. Keep these in a separate area where they can fill the bed themselves or jostle with other strong characters for space.

RAISED BEDS

These allow you to offer herbs better soil and drainage than they would find at ground level, but they also offer advantages beyond the practical. Their straight lines add control to the billow of herbs within, and the extra height garners atten-

tion. They also raise herbs closer to nose level for easy sampling, and are thus convenient for those of us with limited mobility, because they reduce the need for stooping and kneeling.

Most herbs will decline quickly when they are surrounded by dense, wet soil. If your garden is plagued with heavy clay or other slow-to-drain soil, consider lifting your herbs out of harm's way. Building a raised bed for them can solve the drainage difficulties of most herbs, as their roots will usually go no deeper than 15 cm. This means you can create plenty of extra gardening space on top of a driveway, patio or other paving.

To make a frame, use decay-resistant landscaping timbers, anchoring the corners with sturdy metal supports available at DIY and

Unrestrained herbs create a lush composition, weaving together to make a garden seem long-established

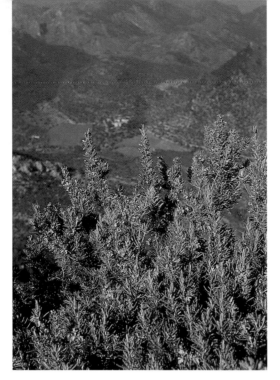

Aromatic rosemary thrives in the kind of arid mountainside conditions that leave most plants gasping for moisture

COTTAGE GARDENS

The romance of an old-fashioned cottage garden goes hand in hand with herbs, many of which have been at home for centuries in humble, country gardens. Recreate the ambience by adding self-sowing herbs that will return year after year to find their place in amongst your flowers.

Some herbs seed themselves so freely that they can become pests in a planned garden. But in the informal, ever-changing style of the cottage garden, this characteristic is welcomed. Herbs and flowers here need to produce plenty of progeny or they stand no chance amongst the other seedlings springing to life each year. If certain herbs begin to overwhelm the garden, however, pull out or hoe off any unwanted plants.

garden centres. Fill the frame with purchased topsoil or improve your soil's texture by mixing it with liberal amounts of coarse sand, compost, peat moss or other organic materials.

Use a single raised bed to enclose a bunch of kitchen herbs, spotlight favourites or lay out several beds with paths running between them. The space in a raised bed is limited, so plant well-behaved herbs that will not spread too quickly.

ROCK GARDENS

It may look inhospitable to us, but a stony, thin-soiled spot actually feels just like home to many herbs, which thrive in the excellent drainage of a rock garden. The stones also invite roots to grow amongst and under them, where they will remain cool and moist. Their contrasting colour and texture will also make your herbs really stand out.

Choose plants that spread slowly or stay in well-behaved clumps for your rock garden, so that your tapestry of herbs remains as you planned it, instead of being swallowed up by a dominant spreading plant. Look for herbs with grey or silvery foliage – a clue that the plant will thrive in the fast-draining soil of a rock garden.

10 best herbs for cottage gardens

borage caraway chicory dill evening primrose foxglove lemon balm marjoram poppies sweet cicely

formal gardens

The guiding hand is very evident within a formal herb garden, with plants growing in a well-defined space. The simplest formal garden consists of well-groomed beds set off by wide paths and stretches of lawn. Select neatly shaped, slower-growing herbs, instead of those that spread rapidly, to maintain the sense of formality. Surprisingly, formal gardens usually require less maintenance than casual styles because each plant sticks to its assigned place.

A formal style also allows room for creativity – try your hand at planting a herb garden in the shape of a wheel or an intricate knot, or section a rectangular plot into a geometric garden or parterre. If you are planting a low hedge or a knot, turn to small-leaved herbs with a dense branching pattern, which can quickly be trained into shape. Plant your formal herb bed where you can admire it from above, from a deck or high window.

KNOT GARDENS

To weave a fanciful knot from herbs of contrasting colour, begin by planning on paper. Once you have a design that satisfies your eye and shows where each strand of the knot goes, mark the pattern on prepared soil with a hoe and set in the young plants. Try to include at least one contrasting colour: perhaps a thread of red-leaved sage or bright silver artemisia. Plant them closely and trim once a month during the first season to promote dense, compact growth.

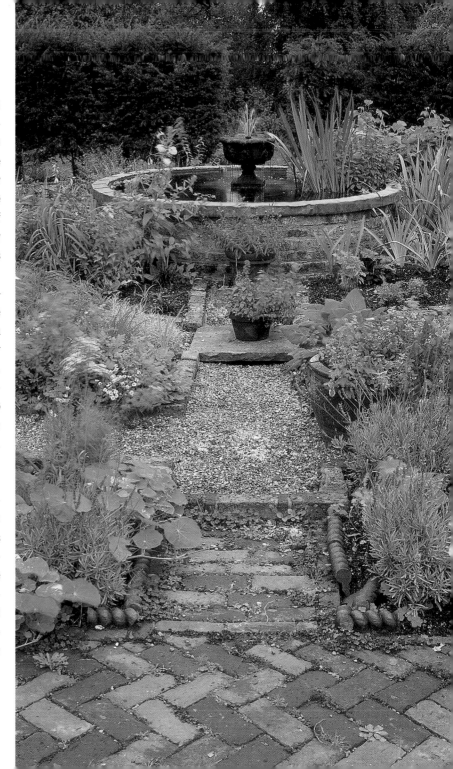

To prepare the wheel garden bed, remove weeds and rake soil smooth and level before laying bricks

Mark segments and scrape out channels in which to lay bricks. Set them in place, pushing them firmly into the soil

Use a pitchfork to work in some gravel to give your herbs the fast-draining soil that their roots will flourish best in

Plant each segment, spacing plants a few inches more closely than the recommended guidelines for a faster finished effect

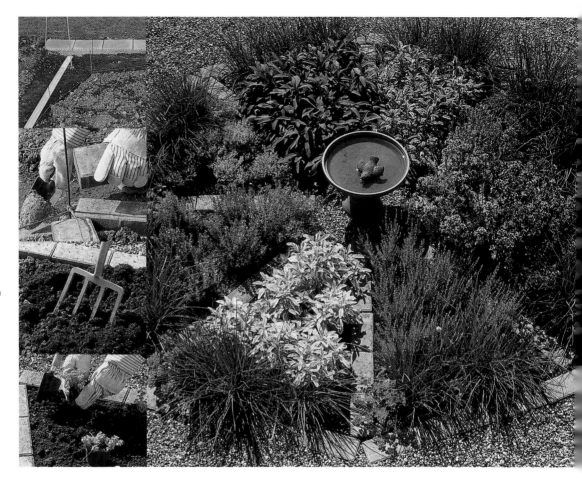

WHEEL

Picture a pie, with each wedge a different herb, and you have the basic form of a wheel garden. You can also dot the centre with a neat, mounded or tall plant, or edge the rim with a low-growing herb such as chamomile. Add definition by edging each wedge with a ground-hugging herb, such as creeping thyme, or lay a flat double row of bricks as the spokes. The wheel design works well for small kitchen gardens, because you won't have to search for your frequently used plants.

PARTERRE

Blocks or triangles of herbs laid within a rectangular or square outline create a parterre. This framework is great to showcase a collection of herbs, such as various varieties of thymes or marjoram. You'll find a symmetrical arrangement, with both halves of the garden mirroring each other in outline, most pleasing to the eye. Use herbs of contrasting foliage colour and texture in alternating segments of the wheel.

The visual strength of straight lines means that even the simplest design, say four intersecting triangles, can be a delight. You can separate each section from its neighbours with a row of brick if you like, or else leave a strip of earth in between to create the borders.

theme gardens

The world of herbs is an extremely large one, with hundreds of possibilities lined up on garden centre tables or tempting you from the pages of a catalogue. Choosing to plan your garden around a particular theme is a great way to focus your exploration by limiting the selection to herbs that fit a certain category.

The choice of theme is entirely up to you – for example, you may decide to start with a sampler of a dozen kinds of thyme, go for various herbs that share a pleasant lemony fragrance or plant herbs that will spice up your favourite style of cuisine. Spend a little time thinking about those aspects of herbs that appeal to you the most, as well as those that you find most intriguing, and use these as a basis upon which to build a theme garden that satisfies your interests.

culinary herbs for worldwide cuisines

ASIAN anise, cardamom, cayenne pepper, lemongrass
MEXICAN cayenne pepper, coriander, garlic
ITALIAN basil, fennel, garlic, marjoram, oregano, parsley, rosemary, thyme
MIDDLE EASTERN cardamom, garlic, parsley, rosemary, saffron
GERMAN chives, dill, horseradish, sage, thyme

CULINARY

A pinch of this, a snip of that, and suddenly even leftovers get a fresh lease of life. Flavour-packed herbs are easy to grow and give you a generous yield even from a single plant. Plant a patch of culinary herbs near your kitchen door and keep a collection in pots on the deck or patio to liven up grilled chicken and other tasty dishes.

MEDICINAL

Backed by generations of folklore, herbal remedies have made a comeback, with bottles of echinacea and aromatherapy potions around every corner. Many medicinal herbs are perfectly safe when used occasionally, but others pack a powerful punch. Whilst there is good reason to be cautious (see page 70), a medicinal herb garden is still a great conversation piece and gives you a feeling of connection to the wise folks of old.

COSMETIC

It's easy to grow the basis for your own soaps, lotions and hair rinses right in your own back garden. Use lavender to perfume a bottle of hand lotion, bring out the highlights in your blonde hair with a splash of chamomile rinse after shampooing or soothe tired eyes with cotton wool dipped in witch hazel. You'll find recipes and tips for making the most of your cosmetic herbs on page 72.

making sense of scented herbs

CITRUSY TANG bergamot, lemongrass, lemon balm, lemon basil, lemon verbena, lemon or orange-scented cultivars of thyme and geraniums
LIQUORICE SCENT anise, fennel, sweet cicely
PUNGENT OR MEDICINAL ODOUR chervil, rosemary, tansy, thyme, witch hazel
SWEET, FLOWERY OR FRUITY AROMA burnet, chamomile, lavender, scented geraniums, sweet woodruff (when dried)

SCENTED HERBS

Delight your senses with a selection of fragrant herbs, arranged to highlight one favourite aroma or as a mixture of perfumes. Even the most fragrant herbs smell only faintly until a leaf is brushed or pinched to release the aromatic oils, so plant your scented garden where the leaves can be easily reached for sniffing.

There are three groups of scented herbs that could form the basis of an entire aromatic garden all by themselves. Cultivars of thyme, scented geraniums and mints carry almost every type of perfume you can imagine, including chocolate, coconut and nutmeg as well as lemon and peppermint. Their foliage and form vary too, so you can make a lovely display from just one group.

GROW A 'FIRST AID KIT'

Try these simple, safe herbs in your medicinal garden:
- Keep a potted aloe plant on the kitchen windowsill and next to your barbecue for quick first aid for burns. Just split a juicy leaf and apply its thick, soothing gel to the skin.
- Sip chamomile tea to calm your senses before sleep.
- Sniff a freshly broken root of horseradish to instantly clear your stuffy sinuses.
- Nibble a leaf of peppermint to quiet an aching tummy. Or quickly remove cooking or tobacco odours from your hands by rubbing the fresh leaves between your fingers.

special places

Because herbs flourish so well in containers, they are perfect for adding a touch of portable greenery to outdoor living spaces like patios, decks and rooftop gardens. Select sun-loving herbs for these gardens, which can take the full force of the sun's rays even when the heat and light is reflected from paved surfaces. Herbs with velvety or fuzzy leaves or foliage that is grey or silver lose less water to evaporation and are well suited for difficult sunny sites.

PATIOS

Bring your garden onto the patio by planting herbs in large pots, wooden half-barrels, formal boxes or other containers. The larger the pot, the less quickly it dries out. Grouping containers also helps reduce evaporation. For minimal watering tasks, plant aloe vera in summer and houseleek, whose succulent leaves hold water in reserve.

Fragrant herbs add an extra sensory pleasure to outdoor gatherings. Culinary herbs are another good choice because you can use them to flavour outdoor meals. Edibles such as tomato or scarlet-climbing beans are other possibilities.

DECKS, BALCONIES AND ROOFS

Plants add a welcoming touch to any outdoor space, giving it the romance of a garden even if there's no soil beneath your feet. Hang window-boxes from the railing of a deck or balcony, or dot a flat rooftop with faux terracotta pots.

You'll want to choose plants that can stand up to heat, light and wind, as well as grow vigorously in a limited amount of soil. Luckily, many herbs are born for such conditions, including favourites such as thymes and lavenders. Coddle your plants by adding water-holding polymer gel beads to the soil mix to ensure a constant source of moisture.

10 best herbs for patios, decks and roof gardens

aloe vera · basil · houseleek · lavender · lemon verbena · marjoram · morning glory · oregano · scented geraniums · thyme

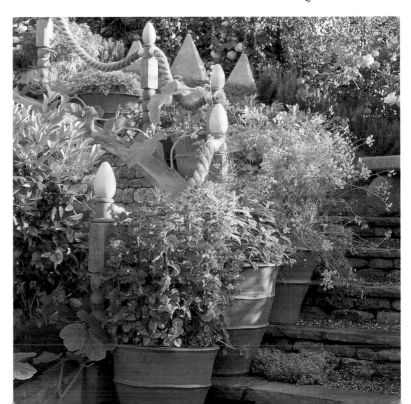

Weight is a big consideration for plants in elevated places – a large clay pot filled with soil can weigh in at 20 kg or more. Stick to lightweight plastic pots rather than heavy terracotta or ceramic, and since herb roots usually stay in the top 15 to 20 cm of soil, fill the bottoms of large pots with non-biodegradable foam packing peanuts. Use a commercial soilless potting mix, which is lighter in weight than topsoil and provides the free drainage that herb roots prefer.

Before you fill your special area with potted herbs, remember that one large container needs less frequent watering than several small ones. Self-watering containers with a built-in reservoir for plants to draw on will also cut down on care.

LAWNS AND GROUND COVERS

Imagine walking barefoot across a swath of springy-soft creeping thyme, each step releasing a fresh burst of scent. It's a lovely image and an easy project to undertake if you use ground-hugging herbs that spread thick and fast. Sprinkle a few flowering herbs into your lawn as well if you like the look; pennyroyal, German chamomile, self-heal and violas will all add colour to your fragrant footing. You can also place stepping stones amongst them if you want to avoid the possibility of wearing a path through your planting.

On steep slopes and other areas where you want to retire the lawnmower, ground cover herbs can do the job, filling in so thickly that they crowd

Plant ground cover in areas among your paving stones. It will spread onto the stones and exude its scent when stepped upon

Prise up your chosen pavers using a sturdy shovel and use a garden fork to mix in coarse sand and organic material

Plant herbs of a dense, low-growing habit, such as creeping thyme or mint, closely together within the allotted space

10 best herbs for ground cover

bergamot   chamomile   creeping thyme   ground ivy   mints   oregano   periwinkle (vinca)   soapwort   sweet woodruff   wild strawberry out potential weed problems. Ground cover herbs can be low growers like creeping thyme that form mats just a few centimetres high, or they may be plants of knee height or more, like bergamot. Look for herbs that expand vigorously from spreading roots, such as mints. In a garden situation, such an aggressive personality is unwelcome, but for covering ground, a tendency to take over is ideal.

Chamomile and creeping varieties of thyme will quickly weave together into a dense lawn, capable of standing up to light foot traffic

LOW HEDGES

A sense of enclosure makes a garden feel cosier, as well as defining areas for various activities. You can use herbs, trimmed or left to grow naturally, to establish low hedges around sitting areas or to guide the eye or the feet from one part of the garden to another. For a taller, more casual hedge, try flowering herbs such as valerian or myrtle, which will form a relaxed row.

Plant herbs for hedges at intervals of about half the recommended distance for garden situations – so that their branches interweave to create a seamless wall. Shear them with electric hedge clippers two or three times a growing season to achieve a neat, formal look and to encourage interior branching.

NICHES

Herbs have a charming habit of snuggling their roots into cracks in paving and other niches. Take advantage of their resourcefulness by starting sprigs in paths and walls to create an appealing contrast to the solid surfaces around them.

Herbs can also hop into inviting cracks all by themselves, sprouting from self-sown seeds. Learn to recognize youthful poppies, thymes and other herbs so that you can appreciate this serendipity instead of mistaking them for weeds.

paths Use a pencil or screwdriver to poke chamomile, woolly thyme and other creeping thymes or low growers into the joints between bricks or stones. Make sure the roots are in contact with the sand between the paving, and spoon a bit more soil over them. Water with a gentle spray and they will quickly grab a roothold. Most herbs rebound quickly from sporadic footsteps, and will also release a delightful scent.

walls Use herbs to spill over the top of walls or wiggle into niches between the layers of stone. Cascading or prostrate varieties of rosemary, creeping thymes and the charming rosettes of houseleeks are good candidates as their roots can fit into tiny niches, finding moisture and sustenance behind the stones. For dry stone walls, built without mortar, use an old butter knife to slide soil into crevices to support the roots.

A screwdriver makes quick work of easing herbs into crevices

the four essentials

Choosing herbs that are at home in your garden is the key to success. Before you invite them in, take time to consider their cultural requirements – soil type, seasonal conditions, humidity and the amount of rain and sun all determine which will grow best.

climate

Your climate is the number-one factor that should determine your choices, although even that is negotiable. Despite the frequent climate-envy felt by British gardeners, there are many techniques, such as growing herbs in pots and wintering them indoors, that will help you to succeed with tender herbs, even in cold-winter areas.

The unpredictable British climate makes it very difficult to advise on particular local conditions suitable for herbs. Even the infamous North–South divide does not always hold true. We have areas in the North warmed by the Gulf Stream and severe frost pockets in the South. Read labels and catalogue descriptions and take a look at the types of plants grown in your neighbours' gardens. The local Horticultural Society can also prove to be a veritable mine of information.

tender and tropical herbs

These warm-weather herbs shiver when freezing temperatures approach. Bring them indoors in early autumn to prevent damage or death from cold: anise, basil, bay, ephedra, hibiscus, lemongrass, lemon verbena, periwinkle, pineapple sage, saw palmetto, rosemary, scented geraniums

Whether a spot is in the sun all day long, or your borders tend to hide in the shade, light should be a crucial factor in your choice of herbs

You can still grow tender herbs in cold areas by enjoying them as one-season plants or by moving them indoors for the winter. If you want to try your luck, you could plant any tender herbs in pots so that they're instantly portable when the weather begins to turn chilly.

As a rule of thumb, you can generally assume that plants that are sold at your local garden centre or nursery will be fairly well adapted to your particular climate. When you start branching out a little and ordering herbs from catalogues and over the Internet, be sure to read carefully the descriptions of recommended conditions and make sure that the plant you want will grow quite happily in your garden.

10 best herbs for shade

angelica   chervil   comfrey   elderberry   lungwort   meadowsweet   periwinkle   self-heal   sweet Joe Pye   sweet woodruff

light

The amount of sun that your garden receives should be an important consideration when choosing your herbs. A sunny spot is the preferred homesite of most herbs, including nearly all the popular culinary types. Many will also grow reasonably well in partial shade, as long as they can bask for at least four hours in full sunlight.

If your garden is a shady one, make those on the list (see page 25) the foundation of your garden, but experiment with others, too. Large leaves are often a signal that a plant will grow happily in most shady situations. Try to avoid planting herbs with grey or silvery leaves in full shade however; they usually decline quickly.

(see page 25)

herbs for problem soils

HERBS FOR ACID SOILS angelica, elderberry, lungwort, senna, sweet woodruff, wild strawberry, witch hazel

HERBS FOR ALKALINE SOILS Austrian briar rose, cucumber, culinary sage, salvias, thymes

HERBS FOR HARDPAN houseleek, mints, oregano, thymes

soil

Herbs are highly adaptable when it comes to soil type. Soil of average consistency will make most herbs happy, but many grow just as well in either light or dense soils. There's no need to bother with a pH test to check the acidity or alkalinity of your soil because these easy-going plants will adapt to all but the most extreme conditions. Rich soil encourages fast, loose growth of foliage, which is usually less aromatic than that of herbs grown on a more meagre diet.

If you can squeeze a handful of earth into a ball that doesn't crumble immediately when you open your hand, or need a crowbar to break it apart, your herbs will have a suitable home. 'Improving'

10 best herbs for dry soils

- aloe vera
- burdock
- fennel
- hemp agrimony
- houseleek
- lavender
- marjoram
- motherwort
- santolina
- **St John's wort**
- vervain

the soil is usually not necessary for herbs. If you have extremely dense clay, however, you can add sand, gravel, compost or other materials to your soil to lighten its texture. Alternatively you can simply select plants to fit your site instead of changing your soil. Herbs with taproots usually do well in clay soil. Because there are so many different herbs to choose from, you're sure to find a number of plants that will thrive in your soil, no matter what its qualities.

Soils that are extremely acid or alkaline, and soils underlaid by an impenetrable rock-hard layer of caliche or hardpan, present special problems for herb gardeners. Either plant varieties that can adapt to these conditions, or make raised beds for your plants. Growing herbs in containers is another way you can expand the possibilities of your herb collection, regardless of the quality of your garden soil.

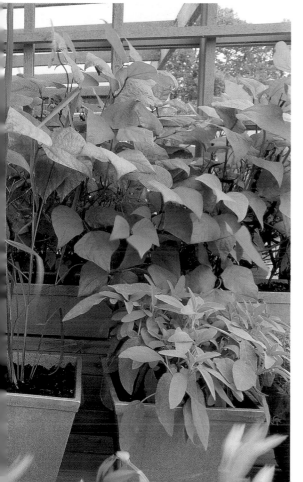

drainage

How fast water drains through your soil is more important to the health of your herbs than the texture or fertility of your soil. Soil that drains slowly, so that the plant roots are frequently in wet soil, will cause most herbs to go into quick decline. Rapidly draining sand and other light soils are usually not a problem, as long as you plant herbs that don't have a thirsty nature.

Compost is a magic cure-all for drainage problems. It fluffs up dense soils, adding air and allowing moisture to pass through easily. It works similar magic on light soils by retaining water that normally dissolves away too soon. Buy or make your compost, and mix it in using liberal amounts.

Growing herbs in raised beds or pots is one way to solve drainage difficulties. You can also select herbs that are adapted to the moisture conditions of your soil. Angelica, bergamot and some varieties of chicory will flourish in wet sites, whilst aloe vera, mallow and burdock like the dry.

Add generous amounts of gravel to clay soils to increase air spaces and improve drainage

preparing and improving the site

You're almost there – now you've thought about what you want to grow and where, it's time to get the bed ready. Preparing a site for herbs is much the same as for flowers, with extra emphasis on giving soil the fluffy, fast-draining soil texture that new roots love.

making the bed

Whilst herbs are generally hardy, adaptable plants, they still benefit from a helping hand and a little groundwork to welcome their new roots.

REMOVING SOD

Peeling up areas of lawn to make way for herbs is a much faster job than you may expect. Grass roots are so interwoven, they will hold together firmly while you roll up your lawn like an old carpet. Here's how to do it:

1 Use a long-bladed digging tool to lift out any dandelions or other deep-rooted weeds.

2 Slice through the turf with a shovel along one edge of the bed – the shorter side, if you're clearing a rectangular area. If your bed is wider than about 50 cm, work in sections.

3 Push the shovel blade in at an angle beneath the edge to sever and lift the first 10 cm of grass roots.

4 Working on your knees, use your hands to begin rolling back the grass. Use a trowel to lift any stubborn spots as you peel up the lawn.

5 Continue until the bed is cleared. Put the sod strips on your compost pile, grass side down.

6 Turn the newly bare soil with a spade, digging at least one blade deep. Chop up any clods using a hoe, then rake smooth.

COMPOST

Rescuing treasure from rubbish is a heartwarming concept for any frugal gardener. Any material that began its life as a plant is fair game for the compost pile: weeds, hedge trimmings, grass clippings, straw, vegetable scraps from the kitchen, newspapers, paper shopping bags – you get the idea. Pile them all up, keep them moist and aerated, and in a couple of months you can scoop out the crumbly black compost from the bottom of the pile.

Earthworms and a million other organisms, from bacteria to beetles, do the work of decomposition by digesting your raw materials. To keep them well fed, aim for a mix of about one part 'green' or fresh plant material to four parts 'brown' or dry plant material. In other words, for every bucket of kitchen scraps you toss on the pile, add four buckets of straw or crumpled strips of torn newspaper. Don't worry about getting the proportions exact; just use your eyes and nose to tell you if the mix is working. If you smell a sour odour, add more dry matter; if the pile doesn't seem to be breaking down, add more fresh green stuff. Avoid any meat, grease or dairy products in the pile, as they will attract pests.

You can build your compost pile within a pen, keep it out of sight in a revolving drum-type container, or just let it grow as a freeform heap. Spray with a hose if rain is scanty so the pile stays moist but not wet.

GRAVEL AND SAND

If your garden soil is heavy, slow-draining clay, a few wheelbarrow loads of gravel or coarse sand will give the roots of your plants better breathing space. Prepare the bed as usual, removing sod and turning the soil. Then dump the sand, gravel or both on top of the new bed. Rake it out to a depth of at least 5 cm, then use a hoe to mix it into the top 15 cm of soil, the depth to which most herb roots will grow.

Be sure to buy washed, coarse builders' sand, not fine-grained play sand, because larger grains are more efficient at improving air and water spaces in clay soil.

Turn over the layers of compost to incorporate more oxygen, which hastens decomposition

choosing plants

Start your shopping with a visit to a nursery or garden centre, where you can see, touch and sniff the plants you've read about. Make a list so you remember to buy at least some of the herbs you've planned space for, but enjoy those impulse buys, too.

When you are faced with so many exciting possibilities for your herb garden, bear in mind the time that you will want to spend on weeding and other care. Lean towards the conservative side when buying – it's always better to start small, and you can always add more plants later.

savvy shopping

Examine the plants closely at garden centres and other outlets before you buy. Always choose the healthiest looking specimens – plants with compact growth, strong stems and no sign of yellowing or other sickliness. If you are ordering through the post, be sure to read the catalogue carefully so that you know what size of plants you are getting, and make sure that the plant will be well-suited for your area.

If you're on a budget or simply enjoy growing your own plants, turn to the seed rack on your herb quest. For less than the price of a single herb plant, you can grow dozens to fill your garden.

As your garden expands beyond the basics, explore the huge selection of herbs to be found in mail-order catalogues and via the Internet – dozens of cultivars of thyme, thirty kinds of lavender... the offerings can seem endless.

2
planting

Treat the new additions to your herb garden with tender care when you settle them into their new home and you'll be rewarded with years of use and beauty. Start with young plants, sow seeds or mix the methods for a lush and bountiful garden.

how to plant your herbs

Herb plants offer instant gratification: you can take them straight home and pop them in the ground. But the cost can mount up quickly. Starting herbs from seed will stretch your budget and give you the pleasure of knowing your herbs from their first sprout.

from the beginning

A few herbs, including popular garlic, are best grown from bulbs. Dill, anise and other annual herbs, which grow for only a single year, are best grown from seed, sprinkled directly into the prepared garden bed. They sprout fast and zoom to a decent size in a short time, outpacing the weeds that infiltrate the bed.

Growing perennial herbs from seed is wonderfully gratifying, and a big money saver if your garden includes more than a few plants of each type. Start perennial herb seeds in pots; the seedlings are tiny at first, and in a garden bed they'd be quickly overshadowed by lusty young weeds. Perennial herbs are slower to sprout than annuals. Most make their appearance in a week or two, but three notorious characters are practically impossible. Leave angelica, lady's mantle, and sweet woodruff to the dedicated experts and plant parsley seed only if you have a lot of patience: it can take months to sprout.

STARTING FROM SEED

Growing herbs from seed can be an almost year-round project, no matter where you live.

• In mild-winter areas, sow seeds for annual and perennial herbs outdoors all year long.

• In colder areas, sow annual herbs directly into the garden during spring, summer and autumn.

When you come to potting your new herbs, fill containers with a lightweight, fluffy planting mix that will resist compaction from repeated watering, confined space and a lack of aerating earthworms. Wet the mix before adding plants

indoors If you live in the north or in a frost pocket, starting perennial herb seeds indoors allows you to get a head-start on the growing season. Sow the seeds about six weeks before you want to move them outdoors. Plant them in pots of soilless seed compost mix and keep them on a tray on a sunny windowsill or under lights. Be sure to label all the pots so you remember what's what! To water, fill the tray with water and let the roots absorb it from the bottom. Apply a water-soluble, all-purpose plant food about once a week.

outdoors Sprinkle the seeds of fast-growing, annual herbs directly into the spot where you want them to grow, following the instructions on the packet to get an idea of how far apart and at what depth to plant them. Most annual herbs will sow their own seeds as the season comes to a close, providing you with the beginnings of a new crop for next year.

You can start your perennial herb seeds in pots outside when the weather begins to get warmer in spring and continue sowing through the early

10 best herbs to grow from seeds

anise basil caraway coriander culinary sage dill German chamomile lavender nasturtium sweet marjoram

Mix very fine seeds with sand to help control the amount you sow. Spray the soil lightly with water and cover with clingfilm to stop the surface from drying out

WHEN TO PLANT YOUR HERBS

agastache	sow seeds from spring to early summer
basil	sow seeds from spring through midsummer
borage	sow seeds from spring to early summer
burdock	plant roots in spring
chamomile	sow seeds from spring to summer
chicory	sow seeds from spring to midsummer
cucumber	sow seeds in late spring through early summer, after soil is warm
dandelion	sow seeds in early spring
dill	sow seeds from spring to late summer
fennel	sow seeds from spring through early summer
foxglove	sow seeds from spring through early summer for bloom the following year
garlic	plant bulbs in autumn
horseradish	plant roots in spring
hyssop	sow seeds in spring through early summer
lavender	sow seeds from spring through early summer for bloom the following year
lemon balm	sow seeds in spring through midsummer
lettuce	sow seeds from very early spring through early summer
morning glories	sow seeds in spring, after soil is warm
parsley	sow seeds from spring through midsummer
poppies	sow seeds in spring. Sow next year's crop in autumn
saffron	plant bulbs (corms) in spring or autumn
sweet cicely	sow seeds from spring through midsummer for bloom following year
tansy	sow seeds from spring through early summer for bloom the following year
yarrow	sow seeds from spring to early summer

summer. After sowing your seeds in a soil-less potting mix, sprinkle a handful of fine gravel on top – this is to help prevent the soil and young plants from being washed away during rain showers. Keep the pots collected together on old trays or baking sheets. Fertilize them about once a week using a water-soluble plant food. When the young herbs have grown large enough to be handled directly and weeded around without damaging their tender new shoots, transplant them into the garden.

If you are sowing seeds or planting roots and bulbs, the guidelines in the chart (left) will help you to grow them successfully in cold-winter areas. In areas where the winters are milder, you can sow and plant year-round. Potted plants are not included – plant these any time during the growing season: year-round in mild climates or spring and early autumn in cold-winter areas. You can also find instructions relating to particular plants in the herb directory (pages 75–187).

STARTING WITH BULBS OR ROOTS

Horseradish, garlic, saffron and other herbs that have bulbous or thick, fleshy roots are usually sold as bare bulbs or roots, although you may occasionally find plants that have already been started offered for sale in pots.

Plant bulbs and roots in spring, summer or early autumn in prepared soil at the recommended depth. Mark the spot with a plant label; it may take several weeks for the shoots to emerge.

STARTING WITH PLANTS

Young herb plants are usually sold in small plastic pots. Make a hole in the bed or container with a trowel, then hold the pot upside-down with one hand across the top to catch the plant as it slips out. If it is reluctant to leave the pot, tap on the base a few times with a trowel until it slides free. Place the root ball in the hole at about the same depth that it was growing in the pot. Fill and firm the soil around it, and water well.

supermarket finds

Shop at the produce counter of your supermarket for economical starts of horseradish and garlic. Look for the gnarled, brown roots of horseradish and the familiar white papery globes of garlic. Store in the refrigerator until you're ready to plant. Separate the garlic cloves and plant individually, about 15 cm apart and 10 cm deep. Plant horseradish roots with the smaller end pointing down, and the top about 5 cm below the surface.

Spring is not just a time for hard work and planting duties, it's also time to enjoy the fresh bursts of floral display your garden will be putting forth

PLANTING CONTAINERS

Containers give you more growing space and serve as focal points in the garden. For the lushest arrangement, fill your windowboxes, clay pots and other containers with as many plants as you can squeeze in. A grouping of herbs of various habits – vertical, mounded and sprawling – will make your container garden more interesting. Soften the look a little with edging plants that will trail over the rim.

After filling the container with potting soil to within 5 cm of the rim, arrange the herbs, still in their original pots, until you are pleased with the combination. Since you will be supplying all the nutrients and water they need, you can plant them closer than you would in the garden.

Water thoroughly after planting. Fertilize with a water-soluble, all-purpose plant food about once a week to keep the plants growing vigorously. Depending on the size of the container and the weather, you may need to water your container garden as often as once a day. Wiggle a finger into the soil; if it feels dry, it's time to water. Fill the container to the brim, let it drain, then repeat.

Be generous when planting containers and snuggle in as many plants as possible. Because you'll be supplying their food and water, they will grow vigorously even in cramped quarters

companion planting

Many gardeners believe that herbs hold the power to deter pests from neighbouring plants, and scientific research into some of the claims shows that there may be truth in this. In any case, it can be fun to conduct your own trials to test the theory in your own garden.

According to some gardeners, it's the strong scent and flavour of herbs that repels pests before they can attack. In some cases, such as garlic and roses, the action is thought to happen above-ground; in others, the repellent is said to be in the herb's roots, for example, marigolds are believed to deter root nematodes.

At the very least, companion planting is a harmless exercise. At best, you may find that combining aromatic herbs with your favourite ornamentals does indeed reduce the outbreaks of aphids and other pests. Keep records so that you can calculate whether such occurrences are due to a general cyclical swing in insect populations, and evident throughout the garden, or if they do seem to be direct cause-and-effect.

PROTECTIVE HERBS

herb	companion	reputed benefits
basil	peppers	enhanced growth
basil	tomatoes	improved flavour and growth
borage	strawberries	improved flavour
borage	tomatoes	encourages bees for pollination
catnip	peppers	aphid repellent
catnip, tansy	potatoes	flea beetle repellent
chives	roses	aphid repellent
dill	cabbage family crops	improved flavour
garlic	roses	aphid repellent
lettuce	radishes	flea beetle repellent
marigold (French)	tomatoes	whitefly repellent
mints	any	ant repellent
nasturtium	cucumbers	cucumber beetle repellent
rosemary, sage	carrots	carrot fly repellent
rue	salad plants	keeps rabbits at bay
rue, wormwood	radishes	flea beetle repellent
sage	cabbage family crops	cabbage butterfly repellent
summer savory	beans	improved flavour
tansy	raspberries	improved growth and better flavour
thyme	lemon verbena	whitefly repellent

attracting beneficial insects

A gardener's best allies against insect pests are other insects – those of a predatory nature, that is. Many species of insects prey upon others, either by devouring them directly or by feeding them to their young. Wasps scour the garden looking for caterpillars to carry off to the nest as a sort of living larder for their offspring. Other wasps lay their eggs on the bodies of caterpillars, upon which the young feed when they have hatched. Ladybird beetles lay their eggs near a colony of feeding aphids so the predatory larvae have a ready-made food source.

These insect allies are known as beneficials. Flowers of dill, fennel and other herbs attract nectaring adult beneficials, which will linger in your garden to work as pest-destroyers.

A range of neighbourly insects benefit gardens by pollinating flowers as they flit between them

10 best herbs for pots

carrot   dill   fennel   garlic   lavender   marjoram   mints   oregano   sage   thyme

tools and equipment

If you already grow flowers and vegetables, you probably have all the equipment needed for working with herbs. A spade, hoe, fork, secateurs, knife and trowel are the basic tools for herb gardening. One other must is labels to help you identify the herbs.

a gardener's toolbox

Well-chosen tools made for the job at hand can make your herb planting and maintenance easy and efficient.

SEED STARTING AND PROPAGATION
A convenient place to work is vital for seed-starting projects. To save your back, work at a potting bench, patio table or kitchen table. A few pieces of simple equipment are all that you need:
• A large plastic cloth to cover the table and make cleanup a breeze
• New or recycled plastic pots
• Soil-less seed compost mix, a lightweight formula that eliminates the problems of compaction as well as weed seeds in normal garden soil
• A bucket for wetting the plant mix, which will take several minutes to absorb the water
• Clingfilm for covering the pots, which speeds the germination process
• Labels to jog your memory and inform guests.

plastic venetian blind labels

Make your own labels from a new, cheap plastic venetian blind (not recycled older models that may contain dangerous toxins). Just one of these should give you a lifetime's supply of labels. Snip each slat into pieces of appropriate length to mark containers or planting beds. Use an indelible marking pen to write the name, then push it in beside your plant.

DIGGING TOOLS

Making holes is how a garden begins, so invest in high-quality digging tools that will stand up to heavy use. Try out the spade before you buy, to make sure its weight and heft are suitable to your strength. Smaller gardeners may prefer a short-handled spade rather than a full-sized handle. Inexpensive trowels are prone to bending and snapping at the neck when put to hard labour in clay or rocky soil. Seek out a trowel with a single-piece blade and handle, made from cast aluminium or other strong metal.

WATERING TOOLS

Herb seeds are often tiny, as are the seedlings that spring from them. A blast of water from the garden hose or even a dousing with a sprinkler can wash seeds far away, or damage delicate roots and stems. Prevent the problem by buying a mist attachment for your hose. This screw-on wand includes a nozzle that breaks the stream of water into a spray of fine, gentle droplets – perfect for seed beds and young herb plantings.

quick connections

Simplify watering chores by buying an inexpensive Y-connector for the tap, so that you can hook up two hoses at once, or leave one side free for filling buckets. Also pick up a screw-on 'shut-off' valve for the tap, so that you can flick a switch to stop the water instead of turning the handle. Your total investment will be minimal. Your total savings in time and convenience will be priceless.

3

maintaining and propagating

Herbs tend to get a lot of attention in the garden, not because they need it – most are trouble-free – but because they're a pleasure to look at, sniff and sample. The shadow of the gardener is the best 'fertilizer' a herb garden can have. Your frequent presence means potential problems will be quickly spotted and solved.

tending your herbs

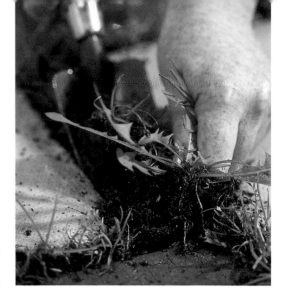

A daily stroll through your garden can make maintenance a quick, casual and enjoyable routine, so that your herbs are vigorous, long-lived and abundant. Take this time to appreciate a moment's calm in the hustle and bustle of daily life.

weed control

These sneaky interlopers compete with other plants for food, water and a place in the sun. Prevent their stealthy thievery by getting rid of weeds whenever you spot them.

Good nutrition is just as vital for young herbs as it is for young humans. If a young herb must compete with weeds for food and elbow room, it is apt to be weak and bare-limbed instead of thick and bushy. If fine work is not your forte, you can eliminate early weeding by sowing seeds in pots, where weeds are nonexistent, or planting your garden from purchased plants.

WEEDING SEEDLING HERBS

Sorting seedling herbs from weeds can be a challenge, but it is also a satisfying exercise, and a vital part of successful gardening. The first step in weeding a new herb bed is deciding which plants are 'keepers'. Determining seedling herbs isn't difficult; a packet of seed will yield dozens of plants that look alike, whereas weeds sprout in all shapes and sizes. And even when very young, herbs carry their characteristic scent. When in doubt, rub a baby leaf and sniff your fingers.

Anise, caraway, coriander and dill are annual plants that germinate and grow quickly, unlike perennial herbs, such as chives, which develop at a much slower rate. Sow annuals thickly and you may not have to weed until the plants are about 5–10 cm tall as they can easily compete with fast-growing weeds. For perennial slowcoaches, weed the bed when herbs are about 5 mm tall, so that they don't get overshadowed by more vigorous weeds. Allow yourself at least an hour to weed, and make yourself comfortable; this is a job to take slowly, so enjoy a moment's calm in the hustle and bustle of daily life.

WEEDING ESTABLISHED HERBS

Weeding around older herb plants is much easier because the plants are so much bigger. There will also be fewer weeds thanks to the shade mature plants create, which discourages germination. Pull weeds whenever you see them, or eliminate them by using mulch or other tricks described. Use a twisting motion to remove older weeds; it will pull roots free with less effort. For deep-rooted perennial weeds, buy an inexpensive 'dandelion digger' – a thin-bladed hand tool to make lifting stubborn roots a simple task.

minimizing weeds

Outsmart weeds by stopping them from sprouting in the first place or by removing them wholesale with a hoe, should they appear. Avoid self-sowing herbs, whose progeny will spring up by the score, unless you are planting an informal cottage garden. Fast-spreading herbs that spread by roots can also run rampant in a tidy garden, but it's usually a simple matter to peel up unwanted mats of plants. Mint is the exception: once this super-fast spreader infiltrates an area, it is difficult to remove because new plants spring up from every little bit of root left in the ground.

USING MULCH

A layer of mulch (see page 44) is your miraculous ally in the battle against weeds. The material prevents sun from reaching weed seeds and also physically blocks their emergence. Grass clippings are an excellent mulch for young weeds because of their fine texture. To get rid of established weeds, use any organic material you have on hand to smother them. If dandelion and other weeds have gone to seed in your grass, avoid using the clippings as mulch to prevent spreading the unwanted seeds.

TOOLS FOR FINE WORK

- Your bare hands are the best tools for this delicate work. Pull out young offending weeds by grasping them between finger and thumb and pulling upwards with a gentle tug. You'll soon develop a rapid, repetitive motion as your eye learns to distinguish weed seedlings from herbs.
- The short, narrow blades of manicure scissors manoeuver easily into tight spaces between seedling plants, allowing you to snip off dozens of weed seedlings with a single motion. Cut close to the soil surface; most will not regrow.
- Regular-size scissors work well for 'teenage' weeds in that skinny, gawky stage when they're 5 to 10 cm tall and still thin-stemmed. Gather a handful together and snip off close to the soil.

Hand weed when herbs are small to prevent competition that could stunt their growth. Mulch older plants with grass clippings or leaves to reduce weeding tasks

Oregano, bergamot, chamomile, creeping thyme and other herbs that spread into thick, dense mats are excellent, living weed-blockers.

mulch

Spreading a layer of organic or inorganic material over soil offers a big pay-off for a small investment. Half an hour spent applying mulch saves you hours of watering, weeding and fertilizing, and keeps your herbs healthy and vigorous. For so little effort on your part, mulch does a lot:

• Keeps the soil from drying out due to evaporation, reducing watering needs.
• Insulates the soil and herb roots within it from the extreme heat of the summer sun.
• Prevents heavy rain from splashing mud onto your herb leaves, keeping them clean for harvest.
• Mitigates winter cycles of freezing and thawing, which damage roots by heaving them upwards.
• Decomposing materials attract earthworms and other organisms that improve the texture of the soil, keeping it loose and light.
• Organic mulch adds nutrients to the soil as it decomposes, increasing its fertility gradually.
• Discourages weeds from getting a roothold amongst your herb plants and makes them easier to pull because of the loose, moist soil.
• Prevents hard rain from washing away soil and exposing the roots of your herbs.
• Helps herbs of borderline hardiness survive cold winters. A deep, loose layer of straw or fallen leaves acts like a cosy quilt.

10 herbs that self-sow prolifically

angelica

borage

caraway

chicory

dandelion

dill

fennel

German chamomile

lemon balm

sweet cicely

WITH CONTAINERS

A single handful of garden soil may contain hundreds of weed seeds. Outwit them by keeping your herbs in containers filled with purchased soil mixes that are free from unwanted seeds. Start slow-growing perennial herb seeds in pots, so they are out of weeds' way for the first several months of their life, or grow an entire collection of herbs in large containers.

DENSE PLANTING

Sunlight is the key stimulant for weed seeds waiting in the soil. When other plants block the light, therefore, few weeds will germinate. Plant your herbs thickly, with little or no space between them, and you'll minimize sprouting of weeds.

GRAVEL MULCHES

Gravel is hard working as well as good looking. It confers most of the benefits of organic mulches, except for bolstering soil fertility. It's a good choice for any area, as it doesn't decompose. Use a 5-cm layer of small-sized gravel, about the size of a pea or smaller, so that weeds can't get a roothold between large stones. You'll find gravel sold at almost all large garden centres and landscaping services. Don't worry if gravel gets mixed with the soil; it helps drainage.

ORGANIC MULCHES

Readily available, sometimes inexpensive (or often free), organic mulches are the most popular choice for garden beds. Use materials from your own garden, like compost or autumn leaves that have been chopped into smaller pieces with a lawnmower. Apply a 5-cm-deep layer over the bed and renew it as it decomposes. Sheets of newspaper make an efficient mulch; disguise it with a layer of more attractive material. For seedlings, apply a thin layer of fine-textured mulch.

Water-soluble fertilizers and foliar sprays encourage vigorous growth of herb foliage

watering

Truly low-maintenance plants, herbs rarely need supplemental water once established, although large-leaved herbs often need more than those with small or feathery leaves. Herbs with grey or silver foliage are usually the least thirsty. Water small seedlings with a fine mist to avoid dislodging roots. If rain is scarce or your plants show signs of wilting, water established herbs with a stronger stream or apply water at their roots with a low-care soaker hose or drip irrigation, which will emit water at soil level and prevent moisture from being lost to evaporation. Spray herb foliage the day before harvesting to wash off any dust or debris that has collected.

fertilizing

A lean diet is not a mean diet when it comes to herbs. Nearly all herbs thrive in soil of average to poor fertility, with many growing well in almost pure gravel or sand, or tiny crevices of soil. Nitrogen-rich fertilizers or manure encourage fast, succulent growth of leaves and stems, which dilutes the concentration of oils that give a herb its characteristic fragrance and flavour.

The best fertilizer for herbs is compost, which supplies a slow, steady, long-lasting nutrient boost. Spread a 2–5-cm-deep layer around your herb plants as a springtime mulch; if another mulch is already in place, use a hoe to pull it back so you can apply the compost to bare soil and then replace the mulch. For tips on making your own compost, see page 29.

winter protection

Hardy perennial herbs, plus any seedlings of self-sown herbs that pop up during autumn, should survive winter in the garden without any assistance from you. To protect tender herbs, there are many ways to pull out the winter blankets: indoors and out.

transplanting indoors

Moving from garden to kitchen window or conservatory is traumatic for herbs used to the outdoor life. Ease the process by beginning early.

1 Younger, smaller plants adapt more easily to indoor culture than established herbs. Instead of trying to move an entire clump of lemongrass, for instance, slice off a small section with a stout knife or sharp spade. Take divisions or cuttings in late summer and root them in 10-cm plastic pots of soil-less potting mix. If

you want to try bringing in an established plant, prune it back by one-third to one-half in early autumn and transplant it into an appropriately sized container.

2 Place the potted herbs in a lightly shaded place, protected from the wind, to mimic the reduced light of the indoor garden.

3 In autumn, before the first frost, check your potted herbs for any pests before bringing them indoors. Place them on a bright windowsill or under full-spectrum or fluorescent lights, and keep them away from heat sources that will quickly dry them out. Supply each pot with a saucer to catch drips; water drains fast through soil-less potting mix, but the roots will absorb the water from the saucer.

4 Be prepared for your herbs to drop some leaves as they become accustomed to the new conditions. Water whenever the soil is dry to the touch 2–3 cm deep.

BOOSTING SURVIVAL OUTDOORS

Get your herb garden fit for the winter season with these preventive maintenance tricks.

• Stop pruning herbs in early autumn so that plants don't produce new growth, which is soft and highly susceptible to winterkill.

• If autumn rains are scarce, water the garden generously before the ground freezes.

• Protect vulnerable perennials like myrtle and bay in cold areas and frost pockets by wrapping in fleece or similar material.

• Move light containers of perennial herbs into a cool or unheated garage for the winter months. Water thoroughly before the soil freezes.

• Snuggle borderline-hardy herbs in a deep layer of straw or loosely piled leaves.

• Lay branches of spruce, fir or any other dense needled evergreens over borderline-hardy herbs when the ground threatens to freeze.

• Treasure snow cover, which has excellent insulation properties. If snow is light and fluffy, you can even shovel it onto any exposed herb plants.

GROWING UNDER GLASS

Savour garden-fresh herbs year-round by growing them under glass. A greenhouse is ideal for keeping herbs through winter, but a simple cold frame will also let you enjoy that fresh-picked flavour.

Enjoy a nibble of fresh herbs with your Christmas dinner by sheltering selected plants with freeze-proof glass covers. Glass domes called cloches – or an overturned clear glass mixing bowl – will help to keep herb plants snug.

quickie cold frames

Solar heat warms up a glass-topped cold frame to keep parsley, rosemary, thyme and other herbs fresh and green, even in cold weather. Kits are widely available or you can construct your own frame from plywood and an old window sash. For an almost-instant cold frame, join four bales of straw into a rectangle and top with a recycled window. Prop the glass top open a few inches on sunny late-winter days to prevent too much heat from building up inside.

pests and diseases

Few insects bother herbs, perhaps because of the substances that create their strong aromas. In fact, herbs are more likely to be pest repellents than fodder for leaf-chomping insects. Disease is also rare and easily managed by non-chemical means.

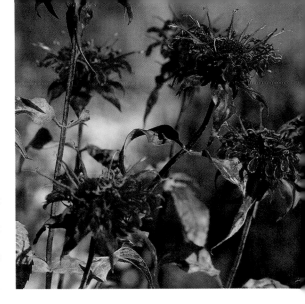

organic controls

Non-chemical methods of controlling pests and diseases solve problems while assuring that herb plants are perfectly safe for you to use in cooking, teas, medicines and other preparations. To maintain a healthy foundation for your herb garden, practise preventive medicine:

a pest with potential

When ridding your herbs of hungry garden pests, bear in mind that you can't have a butterfly without first having a caterpillar! Farming practices and the loss of countryside in Britain threaten many of our indigenous butterflies and moths, so be careful which unassuming little larvae you dispose of, and think about planting some of their favourite foods.

• Keep soil healthy by nourishing the myriad micro-organisms it contains with compost and organic mulches.

• Water your plants early in the day so that foliage dries quickly, thus reducing the potential for mildew and other fungal problems.

• In humid areas, prune back herb plants to keep a bit of space around them for improved air circulation. Damp places are breeding grounds for disease organisms.

• Rotate patches of dill and other annual herbs from year to year so pests don't have a chance to build to problem levels.

• Grow a diverse herb garden. Large areas of a single plant are more inviting to pests.

PROBLEM SOLVING GUIDE

pest or disease	herbs often affected	solution
aphids	caraway, lemon verbena, nasturtium, oregano	snip off infested stems or wipe off aphids with a damp cotton pad
flea beetles	horseradish	lacy, beetle-nibbled leaves are unsightly but harmless to the plant's health. No control is necessary
fusarium wilt	basil	if basil leaves discolour and begin to wilt, pull out affected plants. Plant a new patch with certified disease-free seed in another location
leaf spot	lavender, nasturtium, viola, others	pluck off all leaves showing dark dots and burn or dispose of them in the rubbish bin
mildew	bergamot (see left), calendula, coriander, lemon balm	spray with compost tea made by soaking a shovelful of compost in a bucket of water overnight. Or spray with a mixture of bicarbonate of soda and water
mint flea beetle	mints	cover plants with garden fleece to prevent damage, which is cosmetically unpleasant but not fatal to the plant
scale	bay, rosemary	spray with insecticidal soap or dab a small number of the insects with a cotton swab dipped in alcohol
slugs and snails	all soft leaved herbs	encourage birds, hedgehogs and frogs as much as possible. Create beer traps, and empty them daily. Gravel mulch will also help
spider mites	lemon verbena, mints	encourage beneficial insects by growing dill and other rosemary, sage and thyme herbs with clusters of tiny flowers. Spray plants thoroughly with water, both on the top and the undersides of leaves

Blackfly, a common aphid, tends to cluster on the underside of leaves

Sticky growths of scale like to infest the stems of rosemary and tayberry

The rose chafer, a problem in America, here on a globe artichoke flower, often affects basil

propagation

Making more of a good thing is the reason behind propagating your own herbs. Many plants multiply rapidly with only a little encouragement from the gardener, giving you an abundance of herbs to extend your plantings, share with friends or give as gifts.

10 best herbs to propagate from seed

anise

basil

caraway

coneflower

coriander

dill

flax

German chamomile

lemon balm

rocket

seed

Propagating herbs from seed is so simple you can let your plants do the work for you. All annual herbs produce a generous amount of seeds, many of which will find their way to hospitable soil for next year's crop. If you prefer to direct the process yourself, check the seedheads daily after flowering is finished. When the seeds ripen from green to brown, it's time to collect them.

COLLECTING SEED

You'll need a brown paper bag and a pair of secateurs to collect seed, plus shallow trays for separating seed from plant debris. Harvest only one kind of herb seed at a time, so you don't end up with a mixed bag of seeds.

1 Determine if the seedhead will release seeds when you shake it: Bend the head over the open bag and tap it firmly. If you hear a pattering of seeds following into the bag, continue harvesting in this fashion.

2 If the seeds are reluctant to fall, snip the entire seedhead and let it drop into the bag.

3 Spread the contents of your bag into a shallow tray, such as a clean, empty pizza box. Dry for about a week to ripen seeds.

4 Rub the seedheads between your fingers to release the seeds. Coneflower seedheads are prickly, however, so wear garden gloves.

5 When all the seedheads are cleaned, shake the box back and forth so that the seeds fall to the bottom.

6 Skim the plant debris off the top with your fingers and pour the remaining seeds into a storage container.

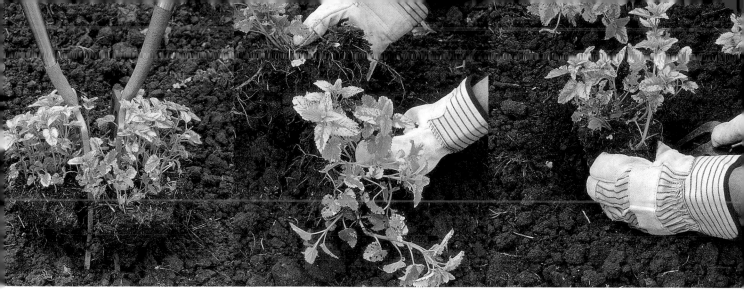

STORAGE AND VIABILITY

Light, heat and moisture are the enemies of stored seeds. Store your collection in small paper envelopes, zip-top plastic bags or closed jars in a dark, dry place. Germination rate tends to be high if the seeds are sown during the first year, but will then decrease progressively with age. If your seeds have been stored for longer than a year, sow them that much more thickly to compensate for their lower viability.

division

Imagine making a dozen plants from a single clump of chives or a hundred new plants of creeping thyme to line a sidewalk. Division is fast and foolproof, and gives you a new generation of good-sized plants within a few short weeks.

Choose herbs with spreading roots to practise on. A spade works best for slicing thickly interwoven roots and stems with little effort. Sharpen the blade with a whetstone beforehand.

SEPARATING SUCKERS

Young plants that pop up near the parent, and spring from the same root, are called suckers. Bergamot, lemon balm, witch hazel and other shrubby herbs often show this characteristic. Use a shovel to slice young suckers from the main plant, then transplant elsewhere. Water well after replanting, and keep the soil fairly moist until they are growing well on their own roots.

Use a garden fork to dig up a large clump of your herb and divide by levering two forks apart

Pull each of the divisions into a further two halves. Repeat if the clump still seems to be too large

Make some new planting holes, add compost and replant the herbs about 30 cm apart. Water well

TIMING

You can divide plants any time from early spring to autumn, but the process is easiest in early spring, when foliage is just beginning to grow and plants can recover quickly from the operation. To divide plants after they are fully grown, cut back the foliage to about 8–15 cm from the ground before slicing up the parent plant.

Remove suckers during the early spring, when the shrubs are still dormant. The transplants will then have more time to grow a few supporting rootlets before they must nourish a whole new growth of foliage.

TECHNIQUE

1 Water the herb plant the day before, so that the moistened soil will cling to the roots, and thus protect the delicate root hairs, when you lift out the divisions.
2 Keeping the blade of your spade nearly perpendicular to the ground, slice through the parent plant, removing a section at least 5 cm in diameter – about the size of a herb plant in a starter pot.
3 Continue slicing off pieces from the parent plant until you have gathered as many divisions as you desire.
4 Replant the divisions in prepared soil and water them generously.

cuttings

Propagating plants by rooting snippets of stem is just as simple as root division, but much less popular, perhaps because it's too tricky to remember which plants will and won't root this way. Lose your hesitation by remembering: 'Nothing ventured, nothing gained'. Try cuttings of any herb you like: if they root, you've gained new plants; if they don't, you've lost only a few minutes' time.

WHEN TO TAKE CUTTINGS

Flexible green stems root faster than tough, woody ones, so take your cuttings in late spring or early summer, when plants put out a flush of new growth. This will allow your plants plenty of time to put out strong roots before winter.

HOW TO START CUTTINGS

A patch of reliably moist soil or sand is all that you need to start cuttings. This soil can be in your garden, where you'll have to contend with weeds and remember to water the cuttings, or in a container, where you can easily monitor growth.

Plastic pots 10 cm or larger in size are ideal for rooting cuttings, because they permit the plant to grow a significant amount of roots before transplanting is needed. Group the pots on a tray where you can water them all at once. A nursery bed dedicated to propagating plants is also a good idea. Mix a liberal amount of compost with the garden soil to lighten the texture so that new roots can easily penetrate and take hold.

TECHNIQUE

1 Examine a healthy, nonflowering stem of the herb you intend to propagate. The bumps from which leaves emerge are called nodes. Using a sharp knife to avoid crushing the stem, slice off a piece about 10–15 cm long, including at least three sets of leaf nodes.

2 Strip the leaves from the bottom 5–8 cm of the stem with your fingers, leaving at least four leaves at the top.

3 If you like, dampen and dip the bare end of the stem into purchased rooting hormone and tap off the surplus. This will speed the root-growing process.

4 Poke the cutting into the moistened soil of the nursery bed or container, pushing it in so that the bare part is all covered. If the stem is very tender, poke a hole with a pencil, insert the stem and firm up the soil around it.

5 Spray the soil with water. Keep very moist but not wet. Cuttings take time to grow roots; keep the soil moist for at least four weeks until new leaves appear. Thereafter, water often, at least once a week if rainfall is scarce.

Run your thumb and forefinger down the bottom of the stem to remove leaves, but keep a few intact at the top of the stem. Push the cutting into the moist soil of your pot and close the soil gently around it

10 best herbs to propagate from cuttings

artemisia   bergamot   hyssop   lemon verbena   mints   rosemary   salvias   scented geraniums   thymes   winter savory

Strawberries are so cooperative that they send out runners with young plants to do the work of rooting for you. Simply sever the rooted plantlets and transplant elsewhere in the garden

layering

This is a propagation technique for the forgetful-minded! You won't have to remember to water, weed or mulch plants. This method takes more rooting time, however – it can take as much as a year before herbs are transplanted to the garden. Try it on any herb you like. If it doesn't work, you've lost nothing and gained knowledge.

TECHNIQUE

1 Select a lower stem that is at least moderately flexible. Gently bend it so that it lies flat at ground level.

2 Where the stem reaches the soil, strip the leaves from about a 7-cm-long section of the stem, keeping the leaves at the stem tip intact.

3 Make a shallow nick in the bare stem on the underside, and slice off a 1-cm sliver of covering or bark – the roots will sprout from here. If you wish to speed up the rooting process, dab commercial rooting hormone on the area from which you stripped the bark.

4 Holding the bare stem to the ground with one hand, mound soil over it and pat firmly into place. Secure with a stone or piece of brick.

5 After weeks or months, depending on the plant, roots will form on the buried stem and the leafy tip will be a separate plant, putting out new foliage and branches. To test progress, pull lightly on the stem tip. You'll feel strong resistance if roots are in place. When well rooted, sever it from the parent just before the buried section and transplant. Water generously for the first few weeks.

10 best herbs to propagate by layering

artemisias bergamot culinary sage elderberry fig lemon verbena rosemary salvias strawberry vervain

4

harvesting, storing and using herbs

Once your plantings are flourishing, you can start to experiment with one of the best parts of having a passion for herbs – making use of them. All herbs are, or have been at some point, employed towards human ends, whether curing nuisance warts, adding a dash of flavour to mash or banishing a musty, lived-in smell. This chapter is designed to give you all the preparatory knowledge you need to liven up your life with a little herb magic.

useful parts

Herbs hold their powers in various parts of their structure. Over the centuries, knowledge of which pieces of each plant are best to use for which purposes has been passed along from generation to generation, as well as from culture to culture.

Foliage is the most commonly used part of a herb, but other pieces of a herb plant may also come into play. Leaves, stems, roots, flowers, seeds, bark and oil – all can be employed, but be sure to pay attention to those parts recommended for use; a tea made from roots instead of leaves, for example, may give unfortunate results.

The method by which the plant parts are prepared is also vital to their use. Some are eaten raw, others boiled or steeped or crushed. Crushed seeds or bark, for example, yield concentrated oils, used for preparations of fennel and some other herbs. You'll find more details on herbal preparations throughout this chapter.

harvesting

Making use of your herbs is an exciting time, whether you're planning to simmer a pot of fresh mint tea or simply to add the colour of some calendula petals to an everyday dinner. You can harvest your herbs whenever you feel that inspiration to liven your home and life with flavour, colour or handmade decorations.

If you need any further encouragement, there is also the fact that the more often you pick, the better your herbs will grow. Cutting herbs causes the remaining stems to push out new branches and leaves, resulting in a vigorous, compact plant ready for further harvest.

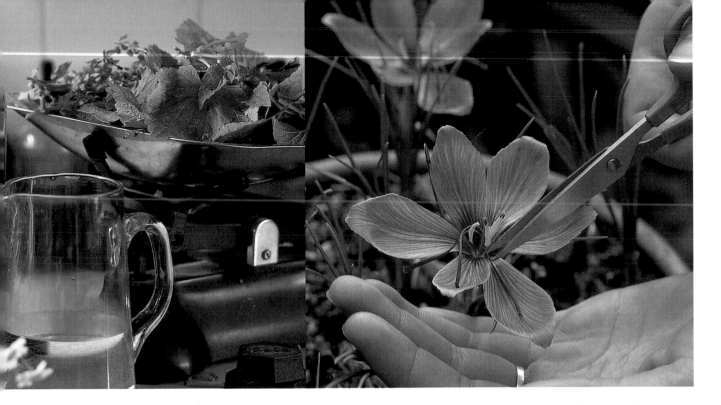

When you pot grow saffron, clip just a few valuable stamens to add colour and flavour to food

COLLECTING LEAVES AND STEMS

Foliage and the stems that it grows on are the parts of your herbs you'll be gathering most – whether you want a sprig of rosemary for roasted potatoes, a basket of basil for summertime pesto or a bouquet of artemisia for future dried flower arrangements. Collect your harvest in whatever container will comfortably hold your treasure. Your bare hand, or a small basket, is fine to carry a meal's worth of seasonings indoors, but if you're picking mint to serve drinks for a family picnic, take a bigger basket out with you. Take care to wash any leaves sprayed with pesticides.

Snip the tender stems of chives, thyme, dill, and other slender herbs with scissors. Secateurs will work better for tough customers like mints, oregano or woody herbs.

when to pick When inspiration strikes, you can harvest your herbs immediately and put them straight to use. If you're planning to store herb foliage, gather it at its most aromatic peak: ideally in mid- to late morning of an overcast summer day, when essential oils are at high levels.

Dry weather generally brings herbs to the height of their aromatic best. After a period of rainy days, the foliage often has a milder scent. In

TIMING THE HARVEST

Gathering herbs is not an exact science. Although flavours and scent vary in strength depending on the season and the weather, you'll still get plenty of your herbs' trademark aromas no matter when you pick.

herb	time to pick	how to pick
annual herbs, including anise, caraway, coriander, dill	any time, as needed; for large quantities, cut twice a season, before flowering	cut entire plant to 15 cm from ground; it will regrow for a second cutting. Snip small amounts any time
basil	repeated cuttings, summer through autumn	cut back each stem until plant is about one-third its size. For last cutting, cut entire plant to ground and use the nonwoody stems and all leaves
bergamot	repeated harvests any time, preferably before flowering	cut back halfway or to ground level
borage	any time when young	snip flowers when blooms are fresh; pick leaves
culinary sage	any time, including after frost, when flavour intensifies	cut tender stems. Avoid cutting into woody part of the plant
garlic	late summer to autumn	dig bulbs at end of growing season
horseradish	autumn	dig root
mints	repeated harvests any time, preferably before flowering	cut back halfway or to ground level
oregano	any time, including winter	snip off as much as desired
parsley	any time, including winter	snip off as much as about half the plant
rosemary	any time, including winter	snip tender stems. Avoid cutting into woody part of plant
thyme	any time, including winter	trim off as much as desired. Only tips in winter

spring, when the foliage is not yet mature, the flavours are usually less powerful. Energy that is diverted to flowers and seed production can also weaken the aroma and flavour of the foliage, so unless you're cutting flowers, harvest your herbs before buds begin to open. In late summer and autumn, herbs may begin to look ragged and insect damage may deface the leaves, but this doesn't mean they're not still tasty!

If you get a hankering for fresh herbs, head outside and snip away no matter what the calendar says. As long as you can find some greenery to snip, you'll enjoy at least a hint of flavour. To avoid stressing the plant, stop snipping perennial herbs from early autumn through the onset of winter, so as not to encourage resource-sapping, new growth at a time when the plant should be slowing down for the colder months.

HARVESTING SEED

Sweet, liquorice-flavoured anise seeds, savoury caraway, sprightly dill and other herbs grown for their seeds are harvested for table use just as they would be picked for sowing a later crop – after they have ripened on the plant from soft green capsules to mature brown seeds holding peak flavour inside.

Monitor your flowering herbs to gauge the ripeness of the seeds, so that the seedheads don't scatter the precious cargo before you have a chance to collect them. To harvest the seeds, shake your seedheads into a paper sack. Pour the collection onto greaseproof paper or a shallow tray so that you can blow gently across them to remove bits of plant debris before storing.

DIGGING ROOTS

The fleshy roots of burdock, chicory, horseradish and angelica and the plump bulbs of garlic are storage organs that hold the collected nutrition of a season's worth of photosynthesis. The plant will draw on this stored food the following year, when new growth begins. Understanding this cycle makes it easy to see that the time to dig herb roots is at the end of the growing season, in autumn. Dig deep with a spade to lift the roots from the soil. If your horseradish patch is a large one, there's no need to uproot the entire thing; just take the roots you need. Shake off any excess soil and wash the roots thoroughly before storing them in the vegetable bin of your refrigerator or drying for later use.

preparing and storing herbs for use

Using herbs fresh is simplest, but you'll also want to put aside a supply for when your favourites aren't available. In long-ago times, air drying was the main technique to preserve herbs. Bunches that are hung to dry still add a quaint touch to the kitchen, but today we can also call upon the microwave, refrigerator and freezer to prepare herbs for storage. You'll find specific tips for each plant in the herb directory (see pages 75–187).

FRESH USE

A quick spritz with cold water to wash off any dust and your herbs are ready to add some pizzazz to the family meals or some fragrance to the bath. For culinary use, you'll also want to remove any tough stems that got into the basket. Mince the leaves or use whole, depending on the herb.

DRYING

The faster herbs dry, the more aromatic they will be. Choose your method according to how much time you want to invest. For herbs used in dried arrangements, air drying is best because it preserves the natural form of each stem.

• Old-fashioned air drying, with herbs hung in loose bunches or scattered on screened trays, is the slowest method of drying herbs; it may take weeks for the moisture to fully evaporate.

10 best herbs for drying

burdock root

chicory root

dill

French tarragon

marigold petals

marjoram

oregano

rosemary

sage

thyme

USEFUL PARTS OF FAMILIAR HERBS

herb	part	use
anise	seed	culinary, medicinal
burdock	root	medicinal
calendula	flowers	culinary, medicinal
cardamom	seeds	culinary, medicinal
carrot	root, seeds	medicinal
cucumber	fruit	medicinal
elderberry	flowers, fruit	culinary
elderberry	flowers, fruit bark, root, leaves	medicinal
evening primrose	flowers, leaves	medicinal
gay feather	root	medicinal
oregano	leaves and stems	culinary
sage	leaves	culinary, medicinal
sweet Joe Pye	flowers, leaves	medicinal
sweet Joe Pye	root	aphrodisiac
thyme	leaves and stems	culinary, medicinal
willow	bark	medicinal
witch hazel	bark, leaves	medicinal

don't even need to chop the herbs before freezing; packed loosely, they will crumble easily in your hand when it's time to add them to a cooking pot. Be sure to label the bag so you can quickly identify it later. You can also freeze chopped herbs as ice cubes: Fill each compartment almost to the top with chives or other chopped herbs, top off with water and freeze. Drop the herb-filled cubes into soups, stews and other dishes.

OILS AND VINEGARS

Combining herbs and oil creates a flavourful additive for pastas, salads and other dishes – or indeed, for softening skin. Use an extra-light olive oil as the base for both culinary and cosmetic magic or try almond oil with sweetly perfumed herbs to flavour desserts. Herb-flavoured vinegars add a savoury touch in marinades, salad dressings and sauces. You'll find intriguing recipes in the herb directory or experiment on your own by beginning with these basic recipes:

• The microwave swiftly speeds up the process, but it requires constant monitoring and frequent reshuffling to dry large quantities (see box).

• A warm oven, set at about 100°C with the door left ajar, is an efficient middle ground, allowing you to process a lot of herbs at one time with minimal fussing. Check your herbs every half hour.

FREEZING

Freezing preserves more of a herb's fresh flavour than drying and it's even easier to do. Buy a box of resealable freezer storage bags and you can store enough herbs for a whole winter of use. You

---

microwave shortcuts

Dried herbs are yours in a flash with a microwave. Ovens vary in power just as herbs do in size and thickness, so experiment with the time you zap each type. Spread herbs of a single kind on a paper towel. Try 30 seconds on medium power and then adjust as necessary. Aim to dry them fully, but not to the point of brittleness, as they may catch fire.

SAVOURY HERB OIL

4 tbsp fresh, chopped herbs, either all one kind
or in combination
500 ml light oil, such as olive or sunflower

Crush herbs with a rolling pin or in a pestle.
Scrape into a bowl and add 2 tbsp oil, stirring to
coat well. Add the rest of the oil and stir well. Pour
into a jar with screw-top lid. Keep at room
temperature for two weeks. Strain the oil into a
bottle with a screw-on top, or pretty jar if a gift.
Add a sprig of herb for a decorative touch. Label
if you like, and store in the refrigerator.

variation For a sweet herb oil to use with fruits
or puddings, use almond oil with chopped leaves
of scented geraniums, lavender or rose petals.

HERB VINEGAR

500 ml white wine vinegar
4 sprigs of culinary herbs, sized to fit bottle
OR
2 tbsp herb seed such as dill, fennel, coriander

Pour vinegar from its original bottle into a fancy
bottle, to about 8 cm from top. Poke in herb sprigs
or pour in seeds. Cap the bottle. Keep at room
temperature for two weeks, then extract herb
sprigs or seeds and replace with fresh ones for
stronger flavour. Store in refrigerator.

10 best herbs for freezing

basil   chives   dill   fennel   lovage   parsley   peppermint   spearmint   tarragon   thyme

putting herbs to use

Herbs were first pressed into culinary use not to enliven the taste of foods, but to disguise it. Before refrigeration, meat was often more than a little 'off' by the time it reached the table, and strong-smelling herbs went a long way towards making it palatable.

culinary magic

Today we use herbs with a lighter hand, enjoying the zing of flavour they bring to favourite dishes. Chicken baked with garlic, for instance, is a savoury dish, while chicken with lemongrass smells equally delicious but has a more sprightly taste. Traditional culinary marriages, like sage with turkey stuffing, oregano in tomato sauces and dill in cucumber salads, have been joined by more adventurous unions. Depend on strong-scented herbs such as garlic, oregano or sage

season to taste

Cooking with herbs is a matter of taste and some experimentation. Use the amounts given in recipes, but if you're cooking freestyle or spicing up a family favourite, restraint is the key – the proverbial pinch between thumb and fingertip will do the trick. Remember, you can always add more, but diluting an overpowering flavour is another story. Basil, chives, parsley, garlic and summer savory become milder with cooking, while French tarragon, oregano, rosemary, winter savory and hot peppers seem to intensify as they permeate the food.

when you're cooking 'heavier' foods, such as meats, soups, stews and tomato-based dishes – meals that require a longer cooking time, under which herbs of a less assertive nature might lose their flavour. For foods cooked quickly, such as eggs, potatoes, rice, stir fries or tofu, try any herb that appeals to you. Salads, cream-cheese spreads, fruit soups and other dishes that need no cooking showcase the full flavour of any herbs.

TEAS

Herbal teas are a guilt-free pleasure. They have no caffeine or tannin, taste delicious and carry no calories. The ritual of tea-making itself and the time spent savouring the drink create a little oasis of calm in which you can indulge yourself.

Fragrant herbal teas are so easy to make from the garden that you may never need to buy another box. A small bed of chamomile or peppermint gives enough flavour for a whole season's sipping, whether you opt for a steaming cup on a winter night or a chilled glass in summer.

You can make teas from fresh herbs at a moment's notice or preserve the harvest for later use. Single-flavour teas are delicious, but it's also gratifying to brew your own custom blends. A base of citrusy bergamot tea, for instance, benefits from the extra tang of lemongrass or rosehips. Or enjoy the unexpected hint of liquorice with a touch of sweet cicely in the mix.

Soothing effects, both mental and physical, are an added bonus, thanks to herbs' medicinal properties. Try peppermint to calm a queasy tummy or unwind with a cup of chamomile after a busy day. Teas from the garden are also great as gifts, costing only a few minutes' time, and earning you brownie points into the bargain.

MATCHING FOODS WITH HERBS

food	complementary herb
beans	summer savory, thyme
beef	garlic, horseradish, marjoram, oregano, rosemary, winter savory
crackers, rolls	dill, fennel, marjoram, oregano, sage, thyme
butter	chives, French tarragon, garlic
butter biscuits	anise, caraway
cakes	anise, caraway, cardamom, lavender, lemon balm, lemon verbena, scented geraniums, sweet cicely
chicken and other poultry	coriander, French tarragon, garlic, lemongrass, lemon verbena, marjoram, mint, oregano, rosemary, sage
coffee	cardamom, chicory
cream cheese	dill, nasturtium, sorrel, watercress
eggs, scrambled	chives, dill, cayenne pepper, French tarragon, lovage, marjoram, oregano, nasturtium, summer savory
fish, crab or other seafood	anise, basil, chervil, coriander, dill, French tarragon, lemon balm, lovage, mint, parsley, rosemary, saffron, summer savory, sweet cicely, thyme
pancakes	anise, chives, sweet cicely
potato salad	chives, dill, parsley, horseradish, marjoram, nasturtium, sorrel, watercress
potatoes, boiled	horseradish, mint, parsley
potatoes, mashed	chives, garlic
potatoes, oven-roasted	rosemary, thyme
rice	cardamom, coriander, marigold petals, parsley, saffron
salad, green	borage, chervil, chives, dandelion, fennel, lovage, nasturtium, sorrel, watercress
sandwiches, meat or cheese	chives, coriander, dill, horseradish
soups, fruit	hyssop, lavender, lemon balm, lemon verbena, sweet cicely
soups and stews	cayenne pepper, chives, garlic, fennel, hyssop, lovage, marjoram, oregano, parsley, summer savory
tofu	lemongrass, rosemary, sage, summer savory
tomato sauce	basil, garlic, marjoram, oregano, parsley, rosemary
vanilla ice cream	lemon balm, lemon verbena, spearmint

bergamot

borage

elderflower

fennel

German chamomile

lemongrass

lemon balm

lemon verbena

mints

rosehip

two ways to brew herbal teas Use a generous teaspoon of dried herbs for each cup of tea. If you're making a larger quantity, figure 1 teaspoon per cup, plus 'a spoon for the pot' – an old saying that gives a slightly richer flavour to steeped brews. For fresh herbs, which are less concentrated in flavour than dried, you'll need 2 to 3 tablespoons per cup. Taste the tea after steeping and add honey or other sweetener if you wish.

RECIPE FOR ONE STEAMING CUP

1 Measure a small amount of water into a kettle and bring it to the boil.
2 Measure dried herbs into a tea ball or home-filled teabag.
3 Fill your cup with boiling water, drop in the container of tea and steep for about 5 minutes.

tea in a teapot Use this method to make a larger amount of hot tea. Measure enough water for several servings into a kettle and bring it to the boil. Meanwhile, measure your chosen herbs into a teapot and press them against the side with the back of a spoon, which will release their fragrant oils. Add boiling water and let the tea steep for about 5 minutes. Pour and enjoy!

ICED TEA FOR ALL THE FAMILY

1 Fill a large or deep saucepan with water and set over medium-high heat.
2 Meanwhile, coarsely chop a generous handful of mint or other fresh herbs, stems and all.
3 Add the herbs to the pan and simmer on a medium heat until you can smell the delicate flavours of the brew. This should take about 5 to 7 minutes.
4 Strain the liquid into a heat-proof container. Discard the herbs.
5 Set the tea aside to cool slightly or add ice to speed the process. This will protect your serving glasses from damage.
6 Fill tall glasses with ice and pour in your custom-made iced tea. Serve it with pride.

EDIBLE GARNISHES

You'll be surprised how much a few green leaves can liven up the appearance of your casseroles or dessert plates. Dress up an everyday platter of pasta with a small bouquet of fresh basil and oregano and your dinner table will instantly be on on the way to that Gourmet Chef look. Nothing but canteloupe for dessert? Make plain melon fancy with a sprig of mint (and maybe a scoop of vanilla ice cream) on the dessert plate.

DON'T GET BUGGED

Insects love the sweet nectar hidden inside herb flowers, but you'll want to be sure not to invite any bugs to dinner. It's easy to pick them from open-faced flowers, but to be sure your edible blossoms are bug-free, treat the insects to a cold chill.
- Put a few blossoms into a zip-top plastic bag. Seal, without pressing out the air.
- Set the somewhat inflated bag upright in the refrigerator for about an hour.
- Insects will flee the flowers to escape the cold or fall out when chilled. They will come to rest on the sides or bottom of the bag.
- After about an hour, carefully remove the blossoms, one at a time, and give them a vigorous final shake, upside down, to dislodge any lingering guests.

Whole fresh leaves, colourful blossoms or even a sprinkling of seeds give meals a finishing touch that makes them look more tempting. All culinary herbs make good garnishes. Select unblemished leaves and flowers. Rinse leaves lightly, but do not wet flowers because their petals may discolour or stick together. Add garnishes just before serving.

• Make herbs of more delicate flavours your first choice, because the idea of a garnish is to complement a food's flavour as well as add eye appeal. A few sprigs of chive blossoms make an oniony accompaniment atop potato salad, more suitable than, say, a spray of liquorice-flavoured fennel, which would overpower the potatoes.

• Choose your garnish according to the flavour of the food. Any herb you use in the cooking will make a palate-pleasing edible garnish. In Italian dishes, for instance, a sprig of basil or oregano will repeat flavours found in the sauce.

• With herbs of medium to large leaves, such as mint or basil, use a snippet of just a few leaves.

• With thyme and other small-leaved herbs, use a bigger sprig or small bouquet so that the garnish stands out visually on the plate.

EDIBLE FLOWERS

Herb flowers bring bright colour to the dinner plate, whether you snip the petals into confetti or use the blossoms whole. Be absolutely sure of your identification before you serve flowers; although the flowers listed here are safe, other garden flowers may cause ill effects when eaten.

10 best herbs for edible flowers

bergamot · borage · calendula · chives · garlic · nasturtium · pansies · primroses · roses · violets

medicinal use

Before the days of modern Western medicine, herbs were used as the cure-all for human health needs, from toothache to nervous conditions, snakebite to childbirth. Ages before Viagra appeared, artichokes and coriander were a man's best friends. And not too many years ago, a dose of chamomile tea, not Ritalin, was the prescription for high-strung children.

Plants have been tested for medical use probably as long as humans have shared the planet. Native Americans chewed willow bark to cure their headaches; today we buy bottles of white tablets – aspirin – containing a synthesized version of the willow's salicylic acid. Soothing teas, invigorating soaks, healing poultices – herbs were the key, whether homegrown or sought from a herbal practitioner. In recent years, herbs have gained great popularity, with medical science working feverishly to test the efficiency of these out-of-the-garden or over-the-counter cures.

The reputed curative powers of herbs are fascinating to learn about, but approach their use with caution. Never rely on an old herbal to treat a medical problem. Experimentation can be fatal. The medicinal strength of herbs varies, depending on weather, climate and soil, so dosage is more guesswork than science. Herbs are powerful plants; monitor yourself for headaches, dizziness, nausea or other side effects. Do not use them daily for long periods and do not experiment with medicinal herbs if you are pregnant. It

is also important that you tell your doctor about any herbal treatments you are taking when you visit for other ailments.

Today some of the same plants once freely dispensed as curatives are known to be poisons. Other herbs have lived up to their folklore reputations when put under the microscope of science. Digitalis, for example, which comes from the foxglove plant, is still the drug of choice for treating certain heart conditions – as it has been used for more than 200 years.

PROVEN TREATMENTS

Under the hard eye of researchers conducting controlled testing, some herbs have been determined to be effective and accepted medical treatments. No one would dispute the efficacy of

While foxglove (right) is too potent to experiment with medicinally, aloe vera (far right) can be made into a safe and extremely effective ointment, or its thick sap can be used straight from the garden to help heal burns and aches

digitalis or aspirin. Aloe is also widely recognized for its skin-healing properties. Still, many herbs have leaped in popularity thanks only to word of mouth rather than formal scientific research.

The worldwide market for herbal treatments has expanded so rapidly that science is hurrying to catch up. While researchers set up tests, consumers are gobbling commercially packaged herbal remedies, currently available without prescription. Clinical trials are under way to test the efficacy of many popular herbal remedies, including echinacea for allergies, St John's wort for depression, saw palmetto for prostate problems, and ginkgo biloba for memory loss. Some countries have reached positive conclusions about these plants; others are still in discussion about their overall effectiveness. Warnings have been

SAFE HERBS FOR COMMON COMPLAINTS

health problem	herb
aching joints	chervil, coriander, thyme
antibacterial, antiseptic	calendula, lavender, lovage, marjoram, oregano, peppermint
bad breath	anise, mint, parsley, sweet cicely
broken heart	borage, viola ('heartsease')
constipation	dandelion, fennel
flatulence	bergamot, caraway, coriander, ginger, lemon balm, lovage, peppermint, summer savory
frazzled nerves	chamomile, dill, goldenrod, lavender, lemon balm
hangover	thyme
hiccups	dill
insect stings	aloe, goldenrod, houseleek, summer savory
insomnia	chamomile, dill
nasal and sinus congestion	horseradish, sage, violet
stomachache, indigestion	dill, fennel, lovage, peppermint
warts	calendula, dandelion, greater celandine

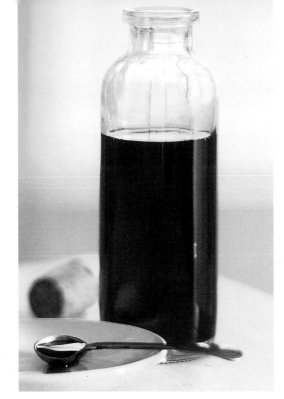

A little dab'll do you when it comes to taking herbal medicines: one single teaspoonful is a common dosage

glossary of medicinal preparations

INFUSION add herbs to boiling water, cover, and steep for about 10 minutes.

DECOCTION boil hard plant parts (seeds, bark, roots) in water for about 10 minutes; steep for 15 to 20 minutes; strain and use.

TINCTURE mix herb with alcohol and add water to reach a 50% alcohol solution; let stand for two weeks, shaking daily, before straining for use.

POULTICE mix dried or fresh herbs with a warm, wet, gluey flour-and-water mixture and apply to skin; wrap with cloth to hold in heat and moisture.

COMPRESS soak a cloth in hot infusion or decoction, wring out and apply.

issued for the once-popular herbal treatment, ephedra, which testing shows can cause strokes, heart attack and other nasty side effects.

PROMISING POTENTIAL

In recent years, more and more plants have gone into the laboratory as scientists experiment with unlocking their medicinal secrets. Collectors scour the world, searching out new plants to be examined for medically valuable compounds and collecting any passed-down folklore remedies that can be tested for their use in modern culture.

Evening primrose is a remarkable recent discovery. Its oil contains gamma-linolenic acid (or GLA), which studies in Great Britain and elsewhere have shown to be effective for treating such disparate conditions as eczema, premenstrual syndrome and even alcoholic hangovers. It has shown promise in more dramatic areas as well: obesity, multiple sclerosis and arthritis.

Madagascar periwinkle is another potential miracle herb, which may be effective in combating cancer. Because modern medicine requires extensive testing to assure efficacy and safety, the time between a trumpeted discovery and its widespread use may form years or even decades. Other herbal cures are likely to be on the horizon shortly, as more and more attention is focused on these age-old helpers of humanity.

home decor

Decorating trends come and go, but there's always a place for herbs in the home. Whether you weave them into wreaths or set them about as potpourri, herbs offer the same benefits indoors as they do in the garden and kitchen: they look pretty, they smell good and they have a soothing effect. Putting your own plants to use in home decoration makes your living space feel more personal, and gives you that wonderful feeling of, 'I made it myself!'

DECORATIVE ARRANGEMENTS

A wire wreath, a spool of florists' wire and an hour or two of time are all it takes to make a beautiful, long-lasting arrangement from home-grown herbs. Try a wreath of culinary herbs for the kitchen wall or add a lavender circlet to the bathroom for a natural air freshener. Dried bouquets are even easier: just insert stems of dried herbs into a block of floral foam inside a basket, vase or other attractive container. Or fill a small vase or glass jar with a simple handful of lavender blossoms on bare stems, dressed up with a raffia or ribbon bow. All the supplies you'll need for herbal home crafts are widely available and reasonably priced at craft shops and garden centres.

It takes a surprising amount of herbs to make a lush-looking arrangement: about 15 fist-size bunches for a 25-cm-diameter wreath, for example. Prepare the herbs by hanging them upside-down in loose bunches to air dry, as described on page 59. If you're more the instant-gratification type, you can also make decorative arrangements with freshly picked herbs and let them dry in place. Because the stems are likely to bend downwards as they dry on the form, monitor your arrangement so you can tuck any strays back into position.

Choose a combination of herbs that pleases your eye. Soft greens and greys can be completely satisfying, or you may want to punch up the arrangement with the deep red of perilla or 'Purple Ruffles' basil, or include a dash of colour from dried blossoms of bergamot, tansy, safflower, calendula or roses.

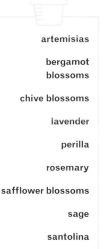

10 best herbs for dried arrangements

artemisias

bergamot blossoms

chive blossoms

lavender

perilla

rosemary

safflower blossoms

sage

santolina

thyme

MAKING A HERB WREATH

1 Measure the circumference of the wreath form in centimetres and divide by ten to estimate how many bunches of herbs you will need. (This allows for overlapping herbs so that 10 cm of foliage is visible from each bunch.)
2 Trim the stems of each bunch to a uniform length, about 15 cm, with secateurs.
3 Lay out a trial circle on your work surface, placing each bunch on top of the stems of the preceding bunch. Rearrange them until you are happy with the combination.
4 Wire the first bunch securely to the wreath form with florists' wire. Cut with tin snips and bend the loose end inside the stems.
5 Lay the next bunch of herbs over the stems of the preceding bunch. Wire the stems of the second bunch into place.
6 Proceed in the same direction with the next bunch and repeat until the form is filled.
7 To cover the stems of the last bunch on the form, insert the stems of a final bunch under the foliage of the first bunch. Wire into place.
8 Hang the wreath and admire your handiwork.

POTPOURRI

It's mystifying how a French word that translates to 'rotten pot' ever came to describe the collection of aromatic materials we think of today as potpourri. Language difficulties aside, a herbal potpourri adds a gentle scent that freshens indoor rooms with natural odours of bergamot, chamomile, lavender, lemon verbena, rosemary, roses, scented geraniums or thymes. With a

Mix spices and essential oils with your flowers, add orris root to make the scent last longer and store in an airtight jar

gardenful of fresh herbs to choose from, you can blend clean-scented lemon mixtures for the kitchen, romantic lavender fragrances for the bed or bath, invigorating rosemary for the office or a host of other possibilities for every room.

Keep your herbal potpourri in a small bowl. Stir the mixture occasionally to release more scent and bring fresher material to the top. Commercial potpourris depend on scented oils that may be artificial or natural in origin. For a longer-lasting and stronger effect, you can add natural oils of lavender, lemon or other fragrances to your mixture. These are available at most herb shops. Alternatively, let the herbs alone perfume your air with a more delicate touch. Orrisroot, a common fixative, helps herbal potpourris last longer too, but with a herb garden at your disposal, you may choose simply to replenish with fresh material as often as you see fit. Dry your herbs for potpourri using any method covered on pages 59–60.

HOW TO MAKE POTPOURRI

1 Strip leaves from selected dried herbs by running thumb and forefinger down the stem. Separate flowers into small florets or petals, depending on size. Discard the stems.
2 Fill container with your herb blend and stir to combine.
3 Drizzle with essential oil and/or fixative if desired. Stir again.
4 Place the bowl on a shelf or table near traffic paths in the house, so passers-by can enjoy it.

CANDLES

Herb leaves and flowers offer appealing shape and colour to the outer surfaces of candles. A simple arrangement is best, so that the scalloped leaf edges, delicate stems or tiny leaves can be best appreciated. Look for candle-making wax, wicks and moulds at craft and hobby shops. Follow the package directions to melt the wax. Before filling the mould with wax, position the herbal decorations. If you like a slightly obscured look, with the herbs peeping through a thin film of wax, pour melted wax into the mould and tilt to coat the sides. Carefully press each leaf or flower into the soft wax. If you prefer the leaves or flowers to be more visible, use tiny dabs of melted wax to anchor each one in place before pouring in the rest of the wax.

NOTECARDS AND PAPER

Speciality papers with petals or leaves pressed into the sheets are pricey but beautiful. Create similar handmade paper yourself.

Fill a blender with crumpled strips of paper, add a cup of water and blend to a soupy liquid. Add more paper, and repeat. Stir in a cup of your chosen plant parts. Pour the slurry onto a framed window screen, and squeegee it into a thin layer. Allow to dry in the sun to slight dampness, then carefully peel the paper off the screen. Flatten the paper using an iron set on medium-high heat, then cut into pieces sized to fit notecard envelopes. Fold, and iron the crease, if desired.

Herbs enliven candles by releasing scent at their base, adding decoration to the wax or providing a delicious scent through extracted essential oils

cosmetic preparations

Your herb garden is a patch of perfumes, just waiting to be used to scent your clothes, skin and hair. While smell alone is enough to calm the senses, herbs can also add shine to your tresses, smooth rough skin, help fight germs with natural antibacterial properties – and, according to some herbal lore, may even stop baldness in its tracks. Using your herbs in home-made cosmetics offers yet another great gift from the garden for birthdays and special occasions.

LOTIONS

Among the easiest cosmetics to cook up at home, skin lotions are simple to make using an inexpensive, unscented shop-bought hand lotion. Buy an economy-size bottle to mix with scented herbs and decant into smaller, more decorative containers that you find in craft shops, catalogues or recycle from your own store of bottles.

LAVENDER LOTION

- Use about 2 tablespoons of dry lavender for each 250 ml of lotion. Bruise the lavender in a mortar or with a spoon, to release as much oil as possible.
- Using a funnel, pour the lavender into the bottle of lotion. Recap and shake well.
- Shake daily for about two weeks.
- Allow the bottle to sit undisturbed for several days, so the herbs can settle to the bottom.
- Stretch a piece of muslin over a funnel and secure with a rubber band.
- Pour lotion from original bottle into smaller containers. The muslin will trap the pieces of lavender, which would be irritating when the lotion is applied.

You can also make water-based herbal lotions to use as astringents, to help clear up skin problems. Calendula is particularly effective for this use. To help dry up pimples, fill a cup of calendula flowers with boiling water, cover and steep for 20 minutes. Allow to cool, then splash onto the face.

SOAPS AND SHAMPOOS

Check craft shops for soap-making supplies and substitute your own herbs for the oils or scents supplied by commercial makers. Rosemary is an excellent choice for hand soap, because its small, stiff leaves provide a bit of abrasive cleaning power and release a sharp, piney scent as you scrub. Lemon-scented thyme and other lemony herbs are ideal for all-purpose shower soaps.

Although you can actually make a lathery shampoo from the herb called soapwort, hair rinses for after shampooing are a better way to take advantage of your favourite herb scents, because you don't rinse them out. Simmer a big handful of lavender, lemon balm, bergamot, chamomile or other favourites in boiling water for about 15 minutes. Strain and cool, and your hair rinse is ready to use. Just pour through your hair after shampooing, then dry and style as usual.

SCENT

Perfume makers use specialized equipment to press the scented oils from herbs, a job that's beyond the reach of home gardeners. But you can

Indulge yourself by concocting your own lotions, soaps and scents direct from the garden – a sensory treat commercial brands just can't match!

still take advantage of the delightful aromas of lavender, thyme and other herbs to add sensory delight to your bath and bed.

For instant relaxation therapy after a stressful day, gather a handful of lavender, chamomile, bergamot or other scented favourites from your herb garden, tie the stems with string and hang from the tap of your bath. As you run your bath, the forceful stream of water will bruise the herbs, releasing their heady scent into the tub and steam. Settle back and indulge!

Make your bed a sensory haven by slipping sprigs of lavender, lemon verbena, rose-scented geranium or whatever herb most delights your nose between the sheets on the shelf. Or tuck a stem of lemon balm or other pleasant-smelling herb directly inside your pillowcase near to the top seam, where the gentle scent will best permeate your sweet dreams.

Pile a loose handful of dried scented herbs in the centre of a cotton handkerchief, collect the corners at the centre and secure the fragrant bundle with a rubber band or tie for a fast and easy sachet to tuck into your drawer of dainty underthings or among your silk scarves. For a fancier sachet, which is suitable for gift-giving, use a square of pretty cotton fabric and fasten it together with a ribbon.

herbs that encourage wildlife

One of the best side effects of planting herbs is the burgeoning number of butterflies and beneficial insects that will soon be attracted to your garden. Most herb flowers are generous with their nectar, the sweet liquid bribe that flowers employ to lure their pollinators. As butterflies, moths, wasps, bees and other insects visit flowers in search of nectar, they become dusted with pollen, which they then unwittingly transfer elsewhere to complete the fertilization of a flower. Mission accomplished, in the perspective of both participants.

IRRESISTIBLE BLOOMS

Red-flowered bergamot, red valerian, thyme, culinary sage and other salvias, are all very attractive to insects. Red valerian will attract the hummingbird hawkmoth in southern England.

Butterflies appreciate the clusters and spikes of small blossoms brimming with nectar on mints, goldenrod and lots of other herbs. Lavender flowers are highly favoured by tiny, dainty blue butterflies. The clustered heads of oregano flowers attract butterflies big and small, which will jockey for feeding space in your herb bed. Painted ladies and peacocks are drawn to the blossoms of purple coneflower, which provide a secure perch for the butterfly while it sips nectar from the many small petal-less flowers that make up the 'eye' of the daisy. Late-blooming goldenrod is a mainstay on the menu of autumn red admiral butterflies.

Adult butterflies are also drawn to herbs and wild flowers that serve as food for their finicky caterpillars, which often eat only one or a very few kinds of plants. Stinging nettles and mallow, for example, are especially popular larval food for the caterpillars of large and small tortoiseshell, painted ladies, comma and peacock butterflies. You may also want to do your bit to boost the numbers of rare and threatened species in your area, and plant the favourite fodder of their particular offspring. In this case, you could contact your local or county wildlife trust for advice on what to plant. Cuckooflowers, for example, will ensure another generation of orange-tips and a mixed group of meadow grass will encourage ringlets, meadow browns and interesting moths.

The more herb flowers your garden offers, the more nectar-seeking visitors you'll attract. But don't worry if your gardening space is limited: even a collection of potted herbs will attract a whole host of butterflies.

10 best herbs for butterflies and beneficial insects

agastache   bergamot   coneflower   goldenrod   hyssop   lavender   marjoram   rosemary   salvias   thyme

5
herb directory

Meet dozens of old, new and unusual herbs in this gallery section, which will introduce you to the personalities, needs and uses of each plant. Throughout the chapter, the planting and cultivation information will address the issue of how to sow or plant each herb. If you are growing from seed, you can assume it is safe to sow directly into the ground outside unless the cultural advice suggests you start in pots. Similarly, pots can be placed either indoors or out, unless specified otherwise.

Achillea millefolium
yarrow

A favourite in perennial gardens, the yarrow grows up to a metre tall. It has an airy feel due to its feathery foliage, which gave it the old name of milfoil, or 'thousand leaves'. The white-flowered species is a pretty plant for borders and cottage gardens. More refined, cultivated varieties bloom in soft salmon, pink, coppery red and pale or butter yellow. All colours give a gentle multi-hued effect, as older blossoms soften to paler shades. One of the longest-blooming perennials, yarrow lends delicacy to larger-flowered companions like coneflower, shasta daisy, irises and roses.

Yarrow flowers add lasting colour to dried wreaths, bouquets and potpourri. The pungent leaves also counteract oily skin or hair; and they help skin abrasions heal. Simmer 2 tbsp dried leaves in 250 ml water and use occasionally to rinse hair, splash an oily face or apply to minor cuts and scrapes. Avoid repeated use, which may cause skin sensitivity or irritation.

planting Grow from seed or buy young plants. Adapts to most soil types; thrives in dry to slightly wet sites. Blooms most in full sun, but also part shade.

cultivation Snip off flowers before they set seed so it reblooms until late autumn. Expands by spreading roots; propagate by division. May self-sow.

harvest Clip flower stems soon after blossoms open; hang to dry. Collect leaves any time for drying on screens; store away from direct light.

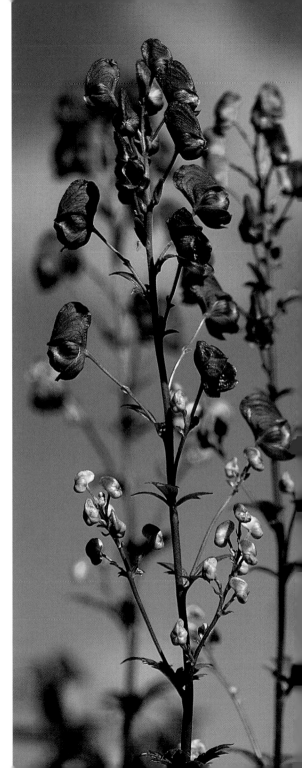

Aconitum spp.
monkshood

Beautiful but deadly even in small doses, this is a herb for remembrance of times past, when the cure could be worse than the disease. Once a poison for wolves and rodents, the plant known as 'wolfsbane' and 'mousebane' may also have been more nefariously employed, as its literally heart-stopping toxin, aconite, works just as dramatically on two-legged animals.

For true-blue colour and vertical height in the garden, this long-lived perennial is a trouble-free (although later blooming) alternative to finicky delphiniums. With stout stems of sharply lobed leaves topped by spires of deep blue, hooded flowers, monkshood may reach almost 2 metres tall, but needs no staking. The emphatic upright form and rich color are a dramatic contrast to asters, eupatoriums, 'Autumn Joy' sedum and other late-season flowers of more relaxed personality. Grow monkshood in ornamental beds, away from edibles, so there is no chance of misidentification and accidental usage.

planting Begin with grown plants; seed is very slow to start. Plant in autumn, in average to fertile soil, full or part sun. Settle top of root just below surface.

cultivation Consider as a lasting garden member; it is long-lived and hard to transplant. Divide the brittle roots every 3 to 4 years. Mulch to keep moist and cool. Grows best if nights remain cool.

harvest Poisonous. Wear gloves and avoid skin contact with all parts of the plant, especially the roots.

Acorus calamus
sweet flag

Resembling a stand of cattails rather than iris, sweet flag flourishes in swamps, streams, lakes and other wet wild places. Its flat, grassy leaf blades shelter an unusual green flower structure that juts out sideways from the three-sided stem, curving slightly upwards. The phallic shape of the flower may have been what caused old-time herbalists to assign aphrodisiac properties to the plant, celebrated in Walt Whitman's erotic 'Calamus' poems. Before you're tempted to experiment with sweet flag yourself, however, be aware that scientific research shows that extracted essential oil distilled from the roots may have carcinogenic properties when it is ingested.

Remarkably, this wetland-loving perennial also thrives in moist garden soil, although it looks most at home planted beside or in a garden pool or pond to add linear grace. Crush a leaf to sniff the spicy-sweet scent; the tuberous roots are also highly aromatic.

planting Start with grown plants. Plant in moist to wet soil, or water, in full to part sun. In smaller water gardens, keep sweet flag in the pot to stop it taking over too much territory via spreading roots.

cultivation Mulch deeply to keep soil cool and moist, if not planted directly in water or boggy soil.

harvest Dig roots in autumn. Dry in a low-heat oven or outdoors on screens. Grind dried roots in blender or food processor. Do not use internally.

a soothing potion for the bath

Sweet flag is reputed to banish insomnia and help calm nervous tension. Try this relaxing addition to your before-bed bath; the delicious fragrance alone will help you forget the stress of the day.

3 tbsp dried roots, finely ground
1 litre water

Bring water to boil over a high heat. Stir in ground roots. Boil for about 1 minute, then remove from the heat and steep for 5 minutes. Strain out bits of root. Add the water to a tub of hot bath water, stirring to combine, and then settle in for a relaxing soak.

Agastache spp.
anise hyssop

A delight in all seasons, this perennial is suffused with a liquorice scent. From summer through until autumn, anise hyssop is covered with fuzzy spikes of flowers that attract butterflies, bumblebees and other nectar-gatherers. Its soft blue-purple can partner most colours: try it with high-voltage red zinnias, lemon daylilies or in a cool group of whites and blues. In winter, the dark, branching stems and seedheads stand out like candelabra. For an eye-catching, off-season composition, combine with various grasses, whose waterfall of bleached autumn foliage makes a great winter backdrop for the bare, upright agastache.

Dried hyssop holds its colour, so is ideal in arrangements or potpourri. Leaves make a fresh flavouring in tea, salad and rice dishes. For more adventures, you could try giant hyssop or Korean mint (*A. rugosa*) or Mexican giant hyssop (*A. mexicana*), both good for tea.

planting Very easy to grow, especially as an annual. Start from seed, buy young plants or beg a cutting; roots easily in moist soil. Plant in full sun, in lean to fertile, well-drained soil.

cultivation Short-lived. Divide in spring or start cuttings in summer. Self-sows if seedheads are not removed; transplant seedlings or cover with mulch.

harvest Snip leaves any time, to use fresh or air dry. Cut flowers when they open and hang dry, or chop as garnish. In winter, use stems for tea or potpourri.

Agrimonia eupatoria
agrimony

Also known as 'church steeples' for its tapering spikes of star-like yellow flowers, agrimony is to be found across Europe in dry fields and ditches. If you enjoy walking on the wild side, you may have already made the acquaintance of this plant, whose barbed 'sticktight' seeds are notorious for hitching a ride on passers-by. But don't let this ingenious method of seed dispersal keep you from enjoying agrimony.

In summer, shade-loving agrimony holds delicate wands of yellow above its foliage, bringing colour to green shade gardens, where it combines beautifully with ferns. This perennial herb was held in high esteem as nature's cure for indigestion. Not only did it quiet an acid stomach, it also relieved constipation and soothed aches and pains. Use it to refresh tired tootsies; steep 3 tsp of dried leaves in a cup of water and add to a footbath. Leaves and stems yield a rich yellow dye for wool or cloth.

planting Easy to start from seed or young plants. Plant in partial to full shade, in any well-drained soil.

cultivation Keep away from paths, so its seeds don't grab unsuspecting visitors. Or snip off ripening seedheads and dispose of them to prevent hitchhiking or self-sowing.

harvest Collect leaves any time for drying. For dye, snip off plant at base in late autumn, cut into pieces and simmer several handfuls in a saucepan for about an hour; strain out herbs and add wool or fabric.

Alchemilla mollis
lady's mantle

Surprised to find a popular ornamental parading through a gallery of herbs? Nearly every plant under the sun has been tried for helpful uses and lovely lady's mantle also had its place in the natural pharmacy at one time. Supposedly, it encouraged blood to clot more quickly, making it useful for primitive tooth extractions, during menstrual difficulties or after an unfortunate accident, whether wild animal attacks, border wars or mishaps with the woodcutting axe.

Nowadays, it's safer and faster to call 999, but it's still nice to know that the pretty lady with the velvety leaves and billows of delicate flowers could come to the rescue in times of true desperation. If you want to experiment, mix young leaves in salads for a bitter tang or infuse 2 tsp fresh leaves in 250 ml water to sip during that week of celebrating womanhood.

Make this versatile plant at home in perennial beds and borders, where she will mingle happily with bearded or Siberian iris, Oriental poppies or any other flower needing a soft feminine touch. Try lady's mantle as an underplanting for your favourite rose, or let it spill over the edges of a path or wall. Lady's mantle self-sows prolifically in most regions. Be sure to take time to admire it after rain, when its pleated foliage holds a net of fine, glimmering droplets.

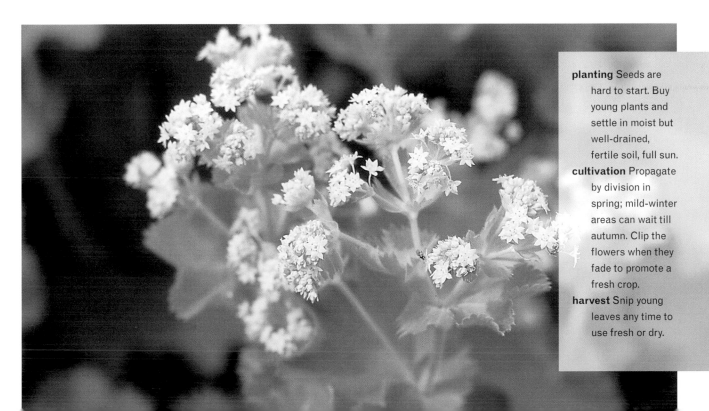

planting Seeds are hard to start. Buy young plants and settle in moist but well-drained, fertile soil, full sun.
cultivation Propagate by division in spring; mild-winter areas can wait till autumn. Clip the flowers when they fade to promote a fresh crop.
harvest Snip young leaves any time to use fresh or dry.

Allium sativum
garlic

Garlic's ability to repel vampires is still open to investigation, but its medicinal successes make an astounding list. Tests have shown it reduces high blood pressure, thus making it a possible aid in preventing strokes. It is also effective at lowering blood sugar levels, an important step towards controlling diabetes. It may help to cure fungal infections, even those that crop up on fingernails and toenails and that are difficult to remedy with modern medicines. Because garlic is reputed to boost the immune system, eating a clove or two a day may help ward off the common cold or flu. With all these benefits, a daily dose of garlic is nothing to sneeze at. So boil the pasta and peel those cloves!

Not only will garlic improve your health, it also livens up your cooking. Its robust oniony flavour has spread from Italian spaghetti

planting Plant in spring or early autumn, in well-drained soil and in full sun. Set individual cloves of garlic, pointed end up, about 10 cm apart and 5 cm deep.
cultivation Apply compost around plants and water regularly for bigger bulbs.
harvest When the tops bend over, usually by late summer, dig up the bulbs and 'cure' on a screen or tabletop for about a week until excess water evaporates and the skin dries to paper. Wipe off soil, cut off roots with scissors and store.

preserving garlic

Each clove you plant will yield a full, plump bulb of garlic at season's end, a bounty that may take you by surprise. Store them loosely in a cardboard box in a dark, dry place, or make a picturesque and time-honoured garlic braid that will keep the herb within easy reach.

1 Consider the bulbs as the top of each strand and the leaves as their bottoms.

2 Lay 3 bulbs side by side and braid their leaves as 3 strands, crossing the left over the centre, right over centre, then left over centre. Repeat the pattern

to gourmet pizzas, roast chicken and even to mashed potatoes – in fact, just about everything but dessert. The intense flavour turns mild with longer cooking, which is why 'Fifty-Clove Chicken' is not a frightening recipe but a mouth-watering one. Whole bulbs are a nutty-sweet treat when roasted; each clove yields a soft pulp that you can squeeze into your mouth.

Snuggle the strappy, dark green leaves of garlic into ornamental gardens, where their pungent odour reputedly deters whiteflies and other pests. Allow easy access for harvesting both the bulbs and the leafy tops, which contribute flavour to eggs, stirfries and other quick dishes. The white or pinkish flowers are also edible. Tone down garlic breath by eating fresh parsley or mint; remove garlic odour from fingers by rubbing mint between them.

Allium schoenoprasum
chives

How bored our tastebuds would be without the fabulous family of alliums! Big brother onion and robust garlic may garner most of the glory, but chives are just as valuable at waking up the flavours of foods and their finer leaves and showier flowers are much prettier in the ornamental garden. Use them to outline a path, to mark corners or to dot a flowerbed with vertical accents. Their pink-purple blossoms appear in late spring and last into early summer, making chives a good companion for the wave of irises and roses that grace the garden at its peak. There's a practical reason for inviting chives into your perennial border, too: like garlic, the aromatic leaves are believed to repel insect pests. If you're fighting aphids and whitefly, therefore, it can't hurt to enlist a crop of these soldiers on your side.

until the braided section is about 5 cm long – the size of a garlic bulb.

3 Lay another 3 bulbs on top of the braided section. Combine the new bulbs' leaves with those of the old bulbs, so that you still have three separate strands.

4 Braid as before until the section is, once more, about 5 cm long. Repeat Steps 2 and 3 until the desired length.

5 Knot the loose ends, trim the excess and hang with the original 3 bulbs at the base. Cut from bottom as required.

planting Start chives from seed in pots, sowing thickly on the surface of moist potting mix; the seedlings look like ultra-thin blades of new grass. Or start with young potted plants. Plant in full sun, in average to fertile, well-drained soil. Also good in pots and on indoor windowsills.

cultivation Water regularly. Cut back hard in midsummer for fresh, new growth. Self-sows, but extras are always welcome.

harvest Snip tops regularly, cutting off just above soil level. Use fresh for best flavour. Cut edible flowers soon after opening. Sniff the blooms – their scent is surprisingly sweet, although their taste is oniony.

Allium spp.
alliums

If you grew up in the country, you may have come across ramsons, the pretty allium to be found in the woods, copses and valleys of mainland Britain. Or perhaps you've detected a garlicky smell after mowing the lawn, as clumps of wild garlic get cut with the grass. Maybe you've seen 'tree onion', with tiny bulbs produced atop its stems. Dedicated flower gardeners may also have played with *Allium moly*, a delicate charmer with liberal butter-yellow blooms, or the huge purple lollipops of

A. giganteum. The genus includes onions, shallots, leeks, garlic and chives, as well as hundreds of lesser known treasures. It's likely that many more alliums share the beneficial properties of some family members, but until the jury is in, explore as ornamental herbs only.

planting Grow from purchased bulbs, as directed.
cultivation Varies according to species.
harvest Keep as flowers unless sure variety is edible.

Aloe vera
aloe

Aloe has been getting good press for thousands of years – and its reputation as a healing herb still holds true today. Ancient armies used it to treat battle wounds, while modern medicine employs it to treat burns from cancer radiation treatments. Soothing and antiseptic, aloe gel heals minor burns, scrapes, cuts and other skin blemishes. Skin mends faster, with less scarring, and pain or itching are instantly relieved. Try it on patches of sunburn, heat rash and mosquito bites, or use it to help clear up acne, dandruff and oily skin.

A tender plant, aloe melts to mush at the nip of frosty temperatures, so keep it indoors or in the conservatory, except in very hot summers, when you can enjoy it as a potted patio plant. Its bold cluster of fleshy, spiky leaves and flowers hold their own by cacti.

No matter where you garden, keep a potted aloe in the kitchen and another near the barbecue, where you can break off a leaf to wipe on any burns from cooking mishaps. The sooner you apply it, the less damage your skin will incur.

Fresh aloe gel is most potent. Simply snap off a piece of leaf about 5 cm long and split with your fingernail to expose the thick, juicy sap. Dab or smear the gel straight onto the skin and let it dry, or use gauze to hold the leaf in place.

Originally hailing from desert regions of Africa, aloe takes in its stride heat, dry air and even lack of water, indoors or out. You can go on holiday with a free conscience, because aloe can go weeks without water, pulling the liquid it needs from its succulent leaves. Give it a generous drink to make its leaves quickly plump up again, ready for use.

---

planting Buy a young plant, or ask a friend for a start. Plant in full sun to light shade, in well-drained soil, in containers. Is an excellent indoor plant.

cultivation Aloe grows fast and needs little care. The plant multiplies quickly, producing 'babies', or offshoots, around the base of the parent. Potted plants flourish even when the roots are crowded. To propagate, pinch off the offshoots and plant each baby aloe in a new pot.

harvest Break off pieces as needed; the broken end will quickly heal over. To obtain larger quantities of gel, break off large leaves at their base, collecting no more than half the leaves from a single plant.

make your own healing potion

1 Thoroughly wash, rinse and dry a small, wide-mouthed jar with a snap-on or screw-on lid. The squat glass jars from speciality mustards, for example, are ideal.

2 Break off about 6 to 10 large leaves from your aloe plant, pinching or else slicing them off at the base.

3 Working on a non-absorbent cutting board, slit a leaf down the centre with a sharp paring knife. Hold the leaf over a small bowl and press the gelatinous juice out of the leaf and into the bowl, using the back of your thumbnail.

4 Slit and extract the juice from the other leaves, working on one at a time. Scrape the collected juice into the jar, using a small, flexible bowl scraper. Label the jar and store in the refrigerator. Apply to skin or scalp as needed.

summer refreshers

On hot summer days, lemon scent is a quick pick-me-up. Try a full menu of lemon verbena: iced tea and biscuits, followed by a citrusy soak or splash.

Steep bergamot and lemon verbena leaves, strain and pour over ice. Accompany with butter biscuits (shop-bought biscuits are a sneaky time-saver), glazed with icing made from 70 g icing sugar, 2 tsp hot milk and ¼ tsp vanilla. Sprinkle finely chopped lemon verbena atop each biscuit before the glaze dries. Afterwards, splash your face with leftover tea diluted with an equal amount of cold water or pour 250 ml into a warm bath.

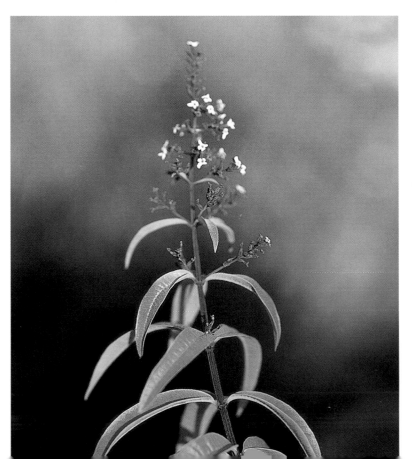

Aloysia triphylla
lemon verbena

The clean, lively scent of lemon is as irresistible in food and drink as it is in cosmetics and room fresheners, so use lemon verbena with abandon in teas, cooking or any herbal craft. Spice up your garden by placing pots near a bench, beside a gate or on the decking, where guests can enjoy the delicious scent of the foliage when they brush against it or reach out and rub a leaf.

This gracefully branched perennial herb is happy in containers and grows vigorously in the garden. Reaching 60 cm tall and wide, with stems that turn woody with age, it makes an excellent anchor for lemon-scented collections. Underplant the willowy-leaved verbena with a mat of diminutive lemon thyme or creeping mother-of-thyme for a pair of pleasing herbs that look and taste good together. Lemon verbena can't tolerate the touch of frost, but it will quickly grow to a good-sized plant in a single garden season, even in cold-winter areas.

planting Seed is difficult to germinate; start with a young plant. Grow in full sun, in well-drained soil.

cultivation Fertilize to boost leafy growth. Water regularly to prevent leaf drop. To overwinter indoors, cut back by about half and move to a sunny window. Propagate by cuttings.

harvest Gather leaves any time for fresh use or drying. Snip leafy branch tip or entire branches. If you don't intend to overwinter the plant, cut at ground level before frost and dry for later use.

Anethum graveolens
dill

Pungent and distinctive in aroma and flavour, this feathery annual herb is as easy to grow as marigolds. Even a single plant produces a bounty of leaves and seeds to add piquancy to main dishes and side salads, and of course to pickles, probably the number one use of dill. Its clusters of tiny flowers will attract beneficial pest-controlling insects to your garden to protect other plants, although it also seems to draw a fair number of slugs and snails, who will munch happily on its ferny greens.

Tall in height but with a delicate personality, dill plants bring a filmy softness to their garden companions. Try a patch of dill with red-hot zinnias or giant lemon-yellow marigolds, or let the self-sown progeny spring up to add airy grace among deep blue salvias and other perennials. For a thoroughly modern use of this time-honoured herb, incorporate chartreuse dill flowers into a modern colour scheme of burgundy-leaved dahlias and lime-green sweet potato vine, or you could use fresh or dried flowers in arrangements.

Dill sprouts and matures quickly, so for a longer display in the garden or a continual supply of fresh 'dillweed', sow in successive plantings, about two weeks apart throughout the growing season. Even seedlings carry the trademark taste, so are good in a simple yogurt-dill dressing for cucumbers or strewn across salmon and other fish.

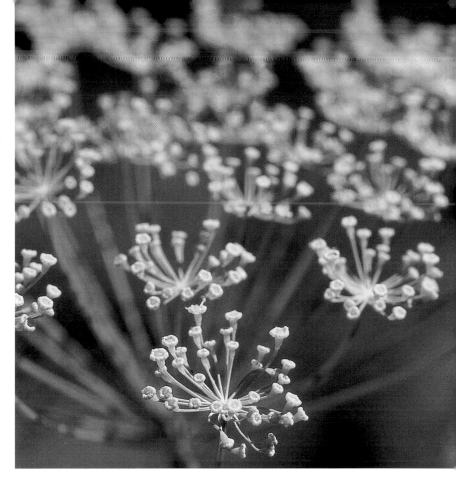

planting Utterly foolproof from seeds sown directly in the garden. Grow in full sun, in well-drained soil.

cultivation Fertile soil or generous fertilizer produces a leafier, taller plant. Clip off seedheads before ripe to prevent self-sowing or smother unwanted seedlings with mulch. Do not transplant.

harvest Cut leaves, flowers and seedheads with scissors. Collect leaves and flowers any time. Use fresh or dried, or freeze leafy stems in zip-top bags and snip, while frozen, into recipes. Shake seeds into a bag and rub seedheads to remove any left.

Angelica archangelica
angelica

Evil witches supposedly steer clear of angelica, whose very name evokes the forces of good. But if you've ever tried to start it from seed, you may have felt ready to side with the sinister instead of the angels. Its reputation as temperamental is deserved, as the seeds lose viability after only a few months. Young plants can be tricky too, because the taproot sulks if disturbed.

It's worth repeated tries to get this statuesque herb into the garden. Its stout, attractive leaves and chin-high stems have a powerful presence, and when the plant blooms, its big greenish-white flowerheads shine across the garden like spotlights. Besides, once you have it, it will crop up year after year as it sows its own successors.

The liquorice-flavoured roots have been used to flavour alcohol, but frequent or large internal doses may cause paralysis of the nervous system – a side effect you definitely want to avoid! The stems are safe to eat sparingly as 'candied angelica', which is simmered in sugar.

planting Buy fresh seeds in late summer or autumn and scatter on prepared soil immediately. Do not cover seeds. Grows in the sun or shade.
cultivation A biennial, angelica forms a clump of big leaves its first year and flowers, sets seed and dies its second year. Learn to recognize seedlings to avoid pulling out self-starters.
harvest Cut the honey-scented flowers any time to make fresh arrangements.

Anthriscus cerefolium
chervil

The subtle flavour of chervil is easy to miss in the rush to fill gardens with familiar favourites. Its understated, slightly weedy form – like an anaemic Queen Anne's lace – doesn't help make it stand out, either. So why grow it? Ask any devotee of French cooking – chervil is a member of the culinary melange called 'fines herbes', valued for adding delicate, fresh flavour to sauces, soups, eggs and cheese dishes.

The flavour of chervil is a hard-to-describe blend of faint liquorice and mild parsley. Some say chervil adds 'warmth' to recipes, perhaps because of that comforting aroma of anise. As a stand-alone player, it transforms steamed fresh peas or ordinary scrambled eggs into culinary bliss. It also is indispensable in the making of any self-respecting béarnaise sauce.

An infusion of chervil may be used in the hope of lowering blood pressure, although this claim is not yet recognized medically. It is also alleged to help prevent wrinkles!

planting Simple from seed scattered on prepared soil. Plant in sun to part shade, in well-drained soil.
cultivation This annual plant matures quickly; sow every two weeks for a constant supply. Pinch or clip off flowers to get a longer harvest of leaves from the plant. Self-sows generously; use unwanted seedlings in cooking and salads.
harvest Collect leaves any time. Use fresh; the delicate flavour quickly diminishes when leaves are dried.

Arctium lappa
burdock

Proving that every plant has a silver lining, burdock leaps from the hedgerow to the herb garden, where you can appreciate the ornamental aspect of its rugged, ruffled leaves as well as the curative power of its root – and then dig it out before it gets a chance to set those prickly round burrs that cling so easily to your pets and clothes.

Burdock is one of many so-called 'weeds' that have made themselves at home in our gardens, either by invitation or by accident. In the case of this herb, it's probably a little of both. Tea made from burdock roots was a popular cure for stomach ailments, so many may have used the plant when there was little else available. The barbed seed coverings have also no doubt been spread tangled in the wool of sheep or other livestock, accomplishing their task of seed dispersal admirably well once they reached hospitable soil.

planting Grows easily from seed. Look for burdock near walls where it escaped the lawnmower or in unused parts of the garden. Thrives in sun or shade.

cultivation A biennial, it remains a ground-hugging cluster of leaves its first year. The next summer, a stem of purple flowers emerges, the seeds mature into brown burr, and the plant dies.

harvest Pick leaves as needed. Dig roots in autumn of the second year, before seeds mature.

quick fix for an itch

Fresh burdock leaves may help soothe the itch of nettle rash, heat rash or even a bad case of mosquito bites. Break off a fresh leaf and crumble it lightly in your hands to bruise the surface and leaf veins. Straighten out the leaf and lay it directly on the irritated skin. Hold the burdock leaf in place for a few minutes, then discard.

Armoracia rusticana
horseradish

One good sniff is enough to test horseradish root's abilities to instantly clear stuffy sinuses. This powerful plant is a member of the mustard family, a large group of plants that share a similar peppery tang. Spurned by animals of the equine persuasion, horseradish gets its name from its coarse, or 'horsey', characteristics. Its thick leaves can grow up to 60 cm long; they form a clump that may measure 1 metre across in less than two seasons of growth and which never stops expanding. Underground, the knobby brown roots may stretch as deep as 60 cm.

As a condiment, horseradish root is unparalleled for adding zing to beef, corned beef, salmon, cream-cheese spreads, potato salad and meat loaf. Mix a bit into mayonnaise-based dressings to give mild-mannered tuna salad or avocados an unexpected spicy bite, or to spread on sandwiches of deli meats or cheeses. Scallops, shrimp and faux or real crabmeat also make a good vehicle for horseradish, either in a white sauce or mixed with ketchup for popular cocktail sauce.

Away from the table, horseradish comes in handy for cold, sinus or allergy problems that make breathing difficult. Just inhale a whiff to clear your head. Its stimulant effect may give some relief to achy or arthritic joints or overtired muscles; spread freshly grated root on a cotton handkerchief and lay on the stiff or sore area.

planting Treat as permanent and give it a corner you won't mind it taking over; it is tough to get rid of once established, as each little piece of root left in the soil will sprout anew. Plant purchased root in sun to part shade, in well-drained soil.

cultivation Mulch to control weeds and keep the soil moist for digging.

harvest Dig roots in late summer to early autumn. Store in the refrigerator to maintain fresh flavour.

two quick & easy horseradish sauces

for sandwiches

1 Peel a 7- to 10-cm piece of fresh root with a sharp paring knife. Grate it manually on a medium to fine grater or else use a food processor.

2 Empty a small jar of commercial mayonnaise into a mixing bowl. Stir in the horseradish one tablespoon at a time, until the spiciness is to your liking. Spoon into a jar and store in the refrigerator. It will keep for months.

for smoked or pickled fish

1 Peel a 2- to 5-cm piece of fresh root with a sharp paring knife. Grate on a medium to fine grater or use a food processor.

2 Combine horseradish, 250 ml low-fat sour cream, ½ tsp Dijon-style mustard, and a pinch of salt. Let the flavours meld for half an hour before serving. Spread on steamed or baked fish, or serve as a side sauce. Also delicious with hot or cold roast beef.

Artemisia spp.
artemisias

Silvery leaves are the hallmark of this genus, a group of aromatic plants that includes wormwood (*A. absinthium*, see upper right), once used in the making of a liqueur whose delirium-inducing effects were immortalized in Degas' painting *The Absinthe Drinkers*. If absinthe isn't your cup of tea, how about vermouth? Wormwood also gave that drink its signature flavour, before the herb's use was outlawed because of its toxic effects.

Strongly bitter in smell and taste, wormwood once enjoyed wide use as a treatment for intestinal worms, a flea repellent and a deterrent to mice and book lice. In a desperate attempt to ward off the Plague, some folks rubbed their bodies with wormwood; although artemisias do have germ-killing properties, wormwood unfortunately can cause severe dermatitis in susceptible individuals.

On the brighter side, artemisias are pretty plants, with billows of pale foliage that can be as fine as lace. Use as hedges, clipped or natural, and as backdrops for white or coloured flowers. The ghostly foliage, held year round in most species, is an effective highlight with red-leaved barberry and other plants of burgundy hue, and with the mellow golds of wintertime, ornamental grasses. The sprays of tiny grey or yellowish flowers (see bottom right) tend to be overshadowed by the foliage.

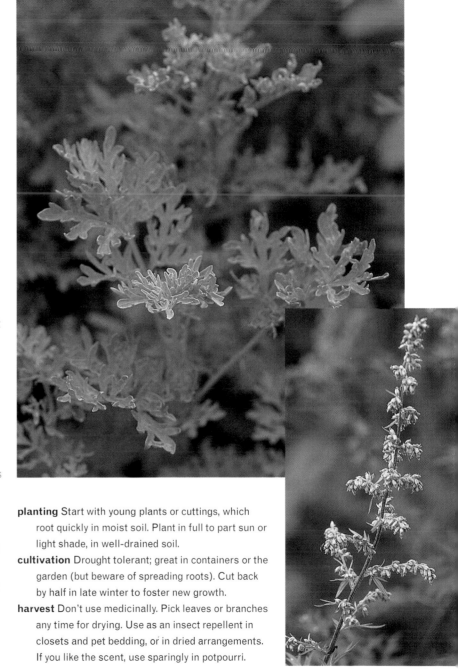

planting Start with young plants or cuttings, which root quickly in moist soil. Plant in full to part sun or light shade, in well-drained soil.

cultivation Drought tolerant; great in containers or the garden (but beware of spreading roots). Cut back by half in late winter to foster new growth.

harvest Don't use medicinally. Pick leaves or branches any time for drying. Use as an insect repellent in closets and pet bedding, or in dried arrangements. If you like the scent, use sparingly in potpourri.

Artemisia annua
sweet wormwood

A fast-growing, highly aromatic annual, with upright green or reddish stems and bright green feathery leaves. Spheres of tiny yellow flowers speckle the foliage in late summer and autumn. Very useful in the herb border to fill gaps or contrast with other, more colourful plants. Sweet wormwood is very popular with flower arrangers, as it dries well, keeping its scent. It is also used for dried arrangements and garlands.

Often found in wasteland across southeast Europe, this herb has also been widely used and well treasured for centuries of Chinese herbal medicine. It was once used to staunch the bleeding of heavy-duty war wounds and to treat conditions as diverse as jaundice, dysentry and skin complaints. Sweet wormwood is also the somewhat unlikely anti-malarial treatment prescribed for the Chinese army, and research has indeed isolated a compound, known as quinghaosu (QHS), which is especially good for drug-resistant strains of the disease.

planting Start with seed, which germinates easily in moist soil. Plant in full sun, in well-drained soil.

cultivation Sweet wormwood does best in dry climates, but feel free to experiment wherever you live as it will thrive in the most unlikely places.

harvest Clip branches or leaves for drying any time, even winter. Use in fresh or dried arrangements, or in potpourri. If the fragrance is pleasing to your nose, slip a sprig of it between wool blankets or jumpers to repel moths.

Artemisia dracunculus
French tarragon

Ordinary chicken salad becomes a speciality of the house when you mix chopped tarragon into the mayonnaise, and fish is sublime with a tarragon-infused sauce. Use it to dress up canned soups or scatter chopped leaves on rice or roasted potatoes. Tarragon turns bitter if it's cooked in dry heat, so use it in sauces or other liquids, or add it near the end of cooking.

If you find yourself nodding off afterwards, you may be experiencing its reputed ability to beat insomnia. Try tarragon tea for a sleepytime treat.

planting Buy a young plant. Tarragon seedlings vary greatly in their aromatic value. Plant in full sun, in light, well-drained soil.

cultivation Do not fertilize; a lean diet makes the flavours more intense. Water container-grown plants regularly, but make sure the potting mix drains quickly; soggy soil will cause a quick decline. Propagate by division in early spring.

harvest Clip leaves and sprigs any time, for fresh use or freezing. Use for flavoured oils and vinegars and in fresh and dried arrangements.

beware of impostors

French tarragon has a strong, complex taste – sweet and lively with a touch of liquorice. *A. dracunculus* subsp. *dracunculoides*, or the lookalike often labelled Russian tarragon, is insipid, with little scent or flavour. Before you buy, rub and sniff a leaf.

Bellis perennis
daisy

Dainty white or rosy pink-edged daisies bloom in early spring with the first dandelions. In mild areas, the charming little flowers may dot the lawn all winter. Although lawn specialists regard it as a weed, this plant can look delightful in a wild flower area or flowering in a natural lawn.

That dainty daisy packs a lot of power in its small blossoms. Made into a tea or infusion, the flowers have been used for generations to heal inflammations and burns, to relieve colds and coughs and as a gentle laxative.

In the garden, English daisies are the perfect companion for early spring bulbs. Try a light or deep pink variety with pale pink hyacinths and silver-and-burgundy ajuga. Let them self-sow between paving stones in walks and patios, or anywhere else they decide to spring up. They are happy campers in container gardens, too, where you can feature their cheerful flowers in a wide, shallow bowl or crowd them around the rim of a big clay pot of blue pansies and white daffodils.

planting Start from seed or buy young plants already in bud. Plant in sun to part shade, in moist soil.
cultivation English daisies have an exceptionally long bloom period, often lasting for several months. For more daisies in the lawn, let the flowers mature into seed before mowing the lawn.
harvest Pluck flowers soon after the buds open and dry for use in teas and infusions.

casual daisies by design
A sprinkling of daisies in the spring grass looks so natural, it couldn't possibly have been planned – could it? Of course it could! Start a patch from a packet of seed in a nursery bed in spring. In autumn, transplant the young perennials into your lawn after the final mowing. Your new daisies will bloom the following spring and for years thereafter.

Borago officinalis
borage

An all-purpose wonder drug in the herbalist's kit, borage is also beloved by beekeepers, cooks and gardeners for its ample, true-blue blossoms.

Medicinal research indicates borage has promise for treating diverse ailments, including arthritis, acne, eczema, fever, premenstrual syndrome and possibly multiple sclerosis. It may also help hangovers and weight loss. Its healing powers are attributed to gamma-linolenic acid, also found in evening primrose. Its leaves add cool, fruity flavour to salads, spreads and dips. The flowers are edible and healthy too, so sprinkle them atop salads or float in a cold fruit soup. To heal skin break-outs, pour boiling water over 500 ml fresh leaves, drape a towel over your head and steam your face for ten minutes.

The large, simple leaves of borage contrast well with plants of finer-textured foliage. Simple from seed, this 60-cm-tall annual makes a pretty partner for chives, shasta daisies, lady's mantle (*Alchemilla mollis*) and pink evening primrose.

flowers in ice

Everyday ice water goes elegant when you add bright blue, starry flowers to the beverage. Instead of floating them in the drinks, where they will interfere with sipping, freeze them in ice cubes. Just drop a pretty borage blossom into each section of your ice cube tray, fill with water, freeze and then serve as usual.

planting Sprinkle seed on bare soil in a sunny site in lean to fertile, well-drained soil.

cultivation Self-sows generously. Smother unwanted seedlings with mulch or plant in a cottage garden. The flowers are beloved by honeybees; keep it away from paths to avoid stings. Annual.

harvest Gather leaves and blossoms any time for fresh use. Chop or slice young leaves for culinary use; steam older leaves for tea or facials.

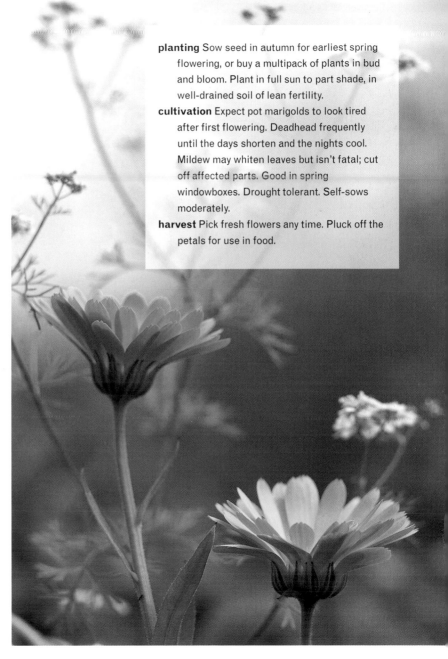

Calendula officinalis
pot marigold, calendula

Contemplating calendulas was a sure cure for the doldrums, said herbalists in medieval times, and who could disagree? The intense golden orange hue of this old favourite is as welcome as sunshine. Within those pretty petals lie healing powers too, because calendula blossoms are antibacterial, antifungal and antiseptic – three properties that make them useful for healing wounds, treating pimples and other infections and making pesky warts disappear.

Calendula petals look just as cheerful in foods as they do in the garden, so use them for a dash of colour in green salads, potato or pasta salads, and soups. Or sprinkle the petals on cake icings for a delightful springtime dessert.

A lover of summer weather, calendula will bloom best from spring to autumn. It will keep blooming even after first frosts, but it rarely lasts all winter. Like the popular daylily 'Stella d'Oro', it has a brassy tint that can be tricky to combine with flowers of other colours. Cultivated varieties of gentler hues are available, but the sunny orange of the species jazzes up the garden and looks great with grey-foliaged herbs. In flowerbeds, choose partners of deep purple, true blue, white, yellow or rusty red. Unless you particularly like clashing colours, avoid planting calendula next to magenta flowers like 'Purple Wave' petunia; use white-flowered or silvery plants between such strong personalities for a less jolting effect.

planting Sow seed in autumn for earliest spring flowering, or buy a multipack of plants in bud and bloom. Plant in full sun to part shade, in well-drained soil of lean fertility.

cultivation Expect pot marigolds to look tired after first flowering. Deadhead frequently until the days shorten and the nights cool. Mildew may whiten leaves but isn't fatal; cut off affected parts. Good in spring windowboxes. Drought tolerant. Self-sows moderately.

harvest Pick fresh flowers any time. Pluck off the petals for use in food.

Capsella bursa-pastoris
shepherd's purse

Many of the weeds growing unnoticed by the wayside are wild plants and escapees from old-time gardens. The common weed called shepherd's purse is most noticeable when its tiny, white flowers have transformed into the spikes of seedpods that give the plant its name. Look closely and you'll see each little pod looks like a three-cornered or heart-shaped pouch, a miniature version of the leather bag holding cheese, bread and perhaps a sip of wine that shepherds would take to the fields.

Shepherd's purse has long been gathered for spring greens, eaten boiled, blanched or raw as a pick-me-up in springtime. After a long winter without fresh greens, this unassuming annual offered a welcome dose of vitamins A and C. Its flavour is mildly peppery, with a hint of cabbage. Herbalists also used the plant to staunch bleeding, encourage labour contractions during childbirth and ease menstrual difficulties.

planting Shepherd's purse may already be growing in your garden. If not, collect seedpods along roadsides and sprinkle on bare soil in full sun.

cultivation Restrict to herb garden to avoid weed problem. Pull self-sown seedlings with a twisting motion, to loosen deep taproot.

harvest Pick fresh leaves in late winter to early spring. Because it may constrict blood vessels, sample only in small quantities, and avoid ingesting this herb if you take blood-thinning medication.

Capsicum frutescens
cayenne pepper

Christopher Columbus first met cayenne pepper in his explorations of tropical America, where it often grows to a height of a metre or more, with a stout, woody trunk. In cold-winter gardens, we know it as a bushy 30-cm-high plant that bears abundant red peppers, then tends to die when the cold weather sets in. This is definitely a plant for your greenhouse or conservatory. Rating quite low on the spiciness scale, unlike the five-alarm habanero, cayenne is perfect for spicing up your chilli, burgers, pasta, eggs and curries.

It is capsaicin that gives hot peppers their heat. Extracted commercially, this substance is used in creams to relieve the pain of shingles and arthritis. Don't try to produce these treatments at home, though, as homemade salves can blister the skin.

Try capsaicin as a pest repellent for garden insects and those greedy squirrels at the bird table: soak a few handfuls of chopped peppers in a bucket of water for 24 hours and spray on plants or birdseed.

Herbalists used cayenne pepper to stimulate the appetite: whether that effect was due to its inherent compounds or to the way it livens up the flavour of food is a question you can research at your own table. More tacos, anyone?

pick a peck of peppers
(pain-free harvesting)

Hot peppers are so powerful they can blister the skin – and you don't even want to think about what happens when capsaicin gets into the eyes. That's why it's essential to handle with care when picking and preparing hot peppers. Cover your hands with rubber gloves, wear a long-sleeved shirt and, above all, resist the urge to scratch an itch on unprotected skin, nose or eyes.

   Also take care when removing the gloves: slip your first ungloved hand into a plastic sandwich bag to pull off the second. The sandwich bag trick is fast and easy when adding hot peppers to food, too; use it to protect your hand when you pull a pepper from the braid or crumble a dried pod into the pot.

planting Sow seed indoors in late winter or buy young plants in late spring. Plant in container or bed of unheated greenhouse for summer.

cultivation Good in containers. May be wintered indoors in bright light. Grow as annual, or as a perennial if you have heat and growing lamps.

harvest Snip off ripe red pods, leaving about a centimetre of stem attached. Spread on screens to dry or string through the stems, using a sturdy needle and carpet thread. Grind to powder in a food processor (wear a mask to avoid inhaling dust).

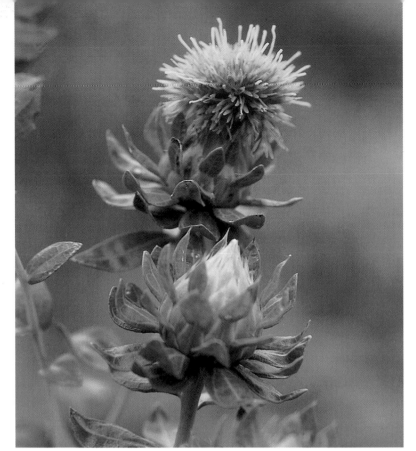

Carthamus tinctorius
safflower

Travel past the dried flower farms in summer and you'll see large areas of safflower glowing deep yellow–orange, like a giant pool of melted butter. In America, massive plantings hold the makings for safflower oil, which has been used by cooks since the days of the Pharaohs. This herb is also prized for attracting butterflies, and birdseed is big business today.

Accent corners of green herb gardens with bright safflower or use it to complement blue salvias or Russian sage (*Perovskia atriplicifolia*). Safflower blossoms keep their colour when dried, so they're perfect for everlasting arrangements. Use the petals to add colour to salads and other dishes, or simmer them in sauces, soups and curries to add a reddish orange tint. The blossoms yield dyes of rich yellow, rusty red and brassy gold, depending on which mordant is used to fix the colour.

safflower silk scarf

1 Buy a lightweight white silk scarf, or finish a length of white silk with a narrow hem.

2 Combine 8–12 litres water and 2–4 litres safflower blossoms in a big saucepan. Bring to the boil, then simmer for about half an hour until the water is intensely coloured. Cool and strain out the flowers.

3 Meanwhile, hand wash the silk in soapy water. Rinse thoroughly.

4 Add the scarf to the dye bath and simmer for an hour. Rinse in very warm water, then cooler water and finally cold water until the rinse runs clear. Hang in the shade to dry, then iron and wear proudly.

planting Sow seed in spring; soak overnight in a saucer of water to speed germination. Plant in a sunny site in lean to fertile soil.

cultivation Tolerates drought. A colourful touch for large containers; try with bright purslane or rose moss (*Portulaca* spp.) for a low-care patio pot. For continued bloom, clip flowers.

harvest Cut flowers soon after they open. Hang to dry, or put in arrangements and allow to dry in place. Inexpensive floral wires, from craft shops or garden centres, can support the flowerheads in bouquets.

Carum carvi
caraway

Caraway and rye bread have been companions for centuries, but the nutty, liquorice tang of this annual or biennial herb also infuses aquavit and kummel liqueurs, as well as sauerkraut, split pea soup and Hungarian goulash. For a quick and savoury side dish, sprinkle halved baked potatoes with Swiss cheese and caraway seeds during the last 15 minutes of baking. In Indian cuisine, the seeds are stirred into dishes and also offered after the meal, both for their palate-cleansing effect and their soothing, flatulence-eliminating properties. The brown seeds are most often used, but the taproot is edible too.

Sow airy, delicate caraway in patches in the herb garden so it doesn't get lost in the crowd of more stalwart plants. Once planted, you'll always have a supply, because some seeds are always overlooked in harvest. These will then plant themselves in various nooks of the garden.

planting Sow seeds in average to fertile soil, in full sun. If you have caraway seed in your kitchen spice rack, simply sprinkle some in the garden.

cultivation Water during dry spells for best flowering and thus more seeds. Pull unwanted seedlings with a twisting motion to free taproot and slice roots in salads or soups. Annual or biennial.

harvest Monitor plants to collect seeds after they ripen to brown but before they fall. Shake into a paper bag, or cut and hang upside down over a cardboard tray; they'll fall out when fully ripe.

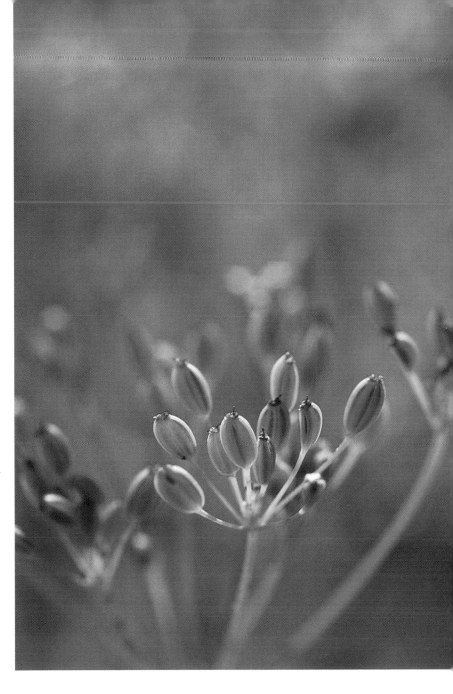

Cassia / *Senna marilandica*
senna

Herbal practitioners have long carried senna in their medicine bags for the same reason you can find it in many over-the-counter remedies today: the plant is a powerful laxative. It's also a striking member of the herb garden, where its unusual foliage and intriguing yellow flowers rise on stems that may reach a metre tall. In winter, the flat, brown seedpods catch the eye and the ear, as they shift and rattle in the wind.

Plant senna to add shrub-like stature to your garden without creating the dense shade of a shrub. This long-lived perennial is also interesting enough to stand alone as a specimen at the centre of intersecting paths. Underplant with golden-leaved thyme or golden oregano to play up senna's yellow flowers in summer.

Homegrown senna is too unpredictable and powerful to use internally, but a mild infusion (1 tsp leaves steeped in 250 ml boiling water for half an hour) may be used as a mouthwash to counteract halitosis and garlic breath.

planting Start with young plants. Plant in well-drained lean to fertile soil, in full sun to light shade. Grows equally well in light, stony soils and dense clay.

cultivation Drought tolerant. Cut back any dead stalks to ground level after leaves appear.

harvest Gather leaves when flowers in bloom, mid-summer to early autumn. Use fresh or dried. For a wall decoration, press a leaf with its oval leaflets in a thick book and mount in a simple frame when dry.

Catharanthus roseus
Madagascar periwinkle

If you live in the South and have a sun-baked spot – along a white masonry wall or house foundation in full sun, for instance – the vivid, abundant flowers of Madagascar periwinkle are just the prescription. This tender perennial soaks up sun and heat, goes without water and never flags. It's understandably one of the most popular bedding plants in recent years.

Eye-popping colours that shine like a spotlight across the garden are another benefit of this adaptable performer. Many cultivars sport dark 'eyes' at the centre of each flower, with white or pastel petals. The foliage is a deep, rich green and the plants fill out into thick, lush growth that knits together into a solid cloak of flower-topped greenery. Bloom begins in early summer and keeps going until frost or through mild winters.

Madagascar periwinkle may prove to be a powerful drug in modern medicines for all kinds of conditions, but this is not a plant to play

modern miracles

Madagascar periwinkle may well turn out to be a miracle drug. The plant contains no less than 60 alkaloids, substances that hold promise for treating many of our most serious health problems. Extracts are already being used to treat childhood leukaemia, testicular cancer and Hodgkin's disease, a cancer of the immune system. It may also hold promise for victims of AIDS and Parkinson's disease.

Because of its powerful approach to slowing growth of tumours, Madagascar periwinkle has similar side effects to other regimens of cancer chemotherapy. It first attracted modern medical attention for its use as a diabetes treatment in Jamaica. Although not in general use, the plant shows some effect at lowering blood sugar in diabetics. It also helps reduce blood pressure.

around with. Even in old herbal lore, it was well respected as a poison, although it was administered in small doses to soothe asthma, consumption, tuberculosis and the common cold. Scientists today are investigating its potential in many varied treatments, from chemotherapy to reducing blood pressure.

Another risky use of Madagascar periwinkle was as an agent to induce euphoria. Unfortunately, the induced feeling of well-being was often followed by serious aftereffects, including death!

Found in hot regions around the globe, the plant adapts easily as an annual in cold-winter gardens. Use it to line pathways, to edge patios and to fill difficult areas with bright colour. It's perfect in windowboxes and patio containers.

planting Buy inexpensive multipacks or potted plants in spring. Can also be grown from seed started indoors in winter. Grow in sun, in well-drained soil of almost any kind.

cultivation No care needed. Blooms continually until stopped by frost. If plants get leggy, cut back by a third to induce branching and compact growth.

harvest Do not use medicinally; highly poisonous when taken internally. Clip stems for fresh bouquets. Snip individual flowers for pressing.

Centranthus ruber
red valerian, jupiter's beard

Too showy to stay in the herb garden, the branching sprays of this perennial herb have migrated to ornamental gardens, where they add a luxuriant splash of colour along paths or in beds with iris, Asiatic lilies and other summer bloomers. Butterfly gardeners also adore this easy-to-grow plant, because its red, pink or white flowers attract crowds of nectar-seekers. Even when not in bloom, red valerian garners attention because its smooth, pale grey-green leaves look so inviting to touch.

The thick, hefty root was once used in herbal remedies for the catch-all categories of 'nervous disorders' and 'hysteria'. Like true valerian, it has a sedative effect. But don't try this at home: an overdose can be fatal and even recommended recipes can have unfortunate effects. Calm your nerves by sniffing the sweet fragrance of the flowers and meditating on the butterflies that dance about the blossoms.

planting Start from seed sown in pots or buy young plants. Plant in full sun, in fast-draining soil. Grows well in lean or alkaline soil.

cultivation Red valerian thrives on adversity. It blooms like mad in gravel and finds every niche in a stone wall. Good for coastal gardens. Self-sows abundantly, often forsaking pampered gardens to spring up in the stony spots it likes best.

harvest Enjoy the fresh flowers in bouquets. Do not ingest the bitter leaves or root.

Chamaemelum nobile
chamomile

Whether you say 'chamomile' or 'camomeal' (both are correct), this herb's name is one of the most familiar to gardeners and nongardeners alike. Good for upsets both physical and mental, chamomile was the remedy for the fevers of malaria along the Nile and the comfort of Peter Rabbit after a run-in with Mr. MacGregor. The demands of modern life keep this calming herb right at the top of any list of favourites.

Two similar but different plants bear the name chamomile: the perennial, ground-hugging species, sometimes called true or Roman chamomile, and a taller annual, also known as German chamomile (see page 138).

Pinch a feathery leaf or squeeze the button of a little chamomile daisy and you'll get a whiff of the clean, fruity scent, reminiscent of windfall apples. That strong aroma was used to

growing between the cracks

Plants snuggled between pavestones and brick gentle a garden with the look of age. Hasten the process by slipping in starts of traffic-tolerant chamomile and thymes. Open a wedge in soil or sand between cracks with a butterknife and push in small, rooted divisions for fragrance in your footsteps.

cover up unpleasant odours in the days before indoor plumbing – strewing the fresh or dried herb on floors created an instant heavy-duty air freshener. While you may not need such strong effects, you can still appreciate the flowers' scent in potpourri or dried arrangements. Or enjoy it in the bath, in sachets or in lotions. For gleaming hair, steep a cup of dried daisies in 500 ml of water and pour over wet hair.

planting Start with young plants, set into well-drained, lean to fertile soil, in full sun.

cultivation Tolerates foot traffic if regularly watered. Transplant into lawns to smell when passing or mowing. To propagate, lift and sever the rooted offsets spreading from the mother plant.

harvest Snip flowers when petals begin to curve backwards, indicating the centre has reached peak flavour. Dry, without removing petals and store in airtight container. Tea or other preparations made from the flowers may aggravate pollen allergies.

cichorium intybus
chicory

Chicory rewards early risers with flowers as blue as the summer sky, but as fleeting as a rainbow: by mid-morning, they have disappeared. This common, somewhat gawky plant is a perennial herb prized for its root and its greens – although both are usually fancied up with an exotic name that hides their origins. The radicchio in the high-priced, speciality greens section of the supermarket and the Belgian endive on your plate at that trendy eatery are both forms of chicory, bred to produce unusual colouring or reliably mild flavour.

Chicory, which is easily invited in, can be difficult to get rid of once settled. Adventurous cooks can cut leaves into shreds to wake up tastebuds with a hint of bitter flavour in salads or stir fries, or contrast the young, tender leaves with sweet mandarin orange segments dressed with a light vinaigrette. To grow a reasonable facsimile of 'Belgian endive', cut a chicory plant to the ground in late autumn, removing all leaves; set an upside-down clay pot over it, cover the drainage hole and in spring, lift the pot to harvest the blanched, emerging shoots.

Chicory was used extensively by early European herbalists, who kept it as a gallstone and gout remedy. The roots, once used as a laxative, are also roasted and ground to make a coffee additive or alternative. Once a favourite in communities of French origin, chicory 'coffee' sometimes received scorn due to unscrupulous nineteenth-century merchants who sold it as true coffee, at high prices. Today, aficionados willingly pay gourmet prices for it.

Combine chicory with red fennel and goldenrod in a meadow planting or cottage garden. Goldfinches and sparrows seek out the seeds in autumn and winter.

french quarter coffee

1 Dig roots in autumn, lifting with a shovel. Cut off side shoots and trim top and tip. Wash well and slice into rounds. Dry in oven at lowest setting, stirring occasionally.

2 When dry, increase heat to 180°C and roast for about 30 minutes, turning occasionally. Cool.

3 Grind in blender or food processor until fineness of the blend matches your usual ground coffee.

4 Brew a pot using about 1 part chicory to 3 parts coffee. Serve with croissants and raspberry jam and imagine yourself on a balcony in New Orleans' French Quarter.

planting Easy to grow from seed, or transplant wild roots to a site in full sun, in well-drained, average to fertile soil.

cultivation Self-sows abundantly; remove unwanted seedlings with a long dandelion digger. Drought tolerant.

harvest Pick leaves young for mildest flavour. Pressed flowers are pretty in crafts; pick soon after opening, in morning. Roots can go 30 cm deep; dig in late summer or autumn. Wash well, trim all but the meaty main section, slice and dry in oven.

Cnicus benedictus
holy thistle, holy ghost herb

Most thistles will fall into the category of horrible garden monster. Even if they don't cause huge invasive problems, thistles can be a literal pain when they escape into the grass, waiting for unsuspecting bare feet.

If it weren't for these tendencies thistles would make wonderful garden plants. Their distinctive, spiny foliage is dramatic in form and texture. The tufted flowers smell sweet, look good and attract butterflies as well as goldfinches, which use the thistledown to line their nests.

The attractive spotted leaves of blessed thistle and its newly flowering tops are edible, despite appearances. The leaves are used for stomach, liver and gallbladder ailments, headache, fever and flatulence. Thistle tea is also occasionally used to stimulate the appetite, and its sharp taste has led to its inclusion in a number of bitters and liqueurs, including Benedictine. Although you may find this annual advertised in catalogues, it's perhaps best to simply admire it from afar.

planting Sow seed in a sunny site, in well-drained soil.
cultivation Grow thistles of any kind only if you are prepared to be vigilant about removing flowers before they set seed.
harvest Collect leaves any time for drying. Clip off flowerheads before they show signs of maturing to form seed puffs.

Coriandrum sativum
coriander

Not too long ago, coriander was usually found languishing in the back of the kitchen spice shelf, the jar of whole or ground seeds pulled out only rarely to sprinkle into the occasional chicken stew. Its infrequent use was likely due to the fact that coriander is a strong-smelling herb, which causes many wrinkled noses at first sniff. The scent supposedly is the same as that of bedbugs, which you'll have to judge for yourself.

As British palates and cooks embraced the flavours of Indian, Asian, Caribbean, Thai, African and Mexican cuisine, as well as plain old meat-and-potatoes, coriander and its green leaves moved to centre stage in the kitchen and herb garden. Now we know a little dab'll do us, this unique nutty, spicy, lemony, musky herb is a welcome addition. Coriander seeds warm the flavour of curries, stews, lamb, chicken, potatoes and gingerbread and other baked goods. Coriander leaves carry a muskier flavour, like sage with a hint of lemon, and taste great with veal, tomato sauces and salads, pasta, corn and eggs. Here is reason enough to dedicate a patch to this simple-to-grow annual herb. But if you need another plus, in the spicy climes of Arabia and dank castles of the Middle Ages, coriander was used as an aphrodisiac.

The tall, open, fine-leafed plants offer clusters of understated white flowers, but tend to flop over as the seeds ripen. Edge with bright red salvia for contrast and informal stem support.

planting Sow seeds in well-drained, average soil, in full sun to part shade, in spring to midsummer. Sow thickly in rows to make early weeding easier. Grow year-round in mild-winter regions.

cultivation Make successive plantings, 2–3 weeks apart, for bountiful coriander.

harvest Pick lower leaves any time for fresh use; finer leaves at the top of the plant have an intense, somewhat unpleasant flavour. Unripe seeds smell bad, but they mature to pleasant lemony maturity. When the plant turns brown, cut at ground level and hang over trays to let seeds drop out when they're ready. Store seed in tightly closed jars; use whole or grind before use.

a must for mexican cuisine

Coriander is the mystery player in Mexican food, that unusual flavour you can't quite identify. Pluck leaves from stems, bruise them in your palms and stir into chicken molé, tomatillo salsa, roasted corn and black bean dip for authentic Central American flavour.

Crocus sativus
saffron

Harvesting this herb will make you feel like you're in a fairy tale: plucking rich orange threads from inside a beautiful purple flower to make culinary magic. You'll feel even more like a fairy-tale character – rich old King Midas – when you consider that saffron is the world's costliest herb. That's because it takes more than a thousand flowers to yield only 25 grams of saffron, and every thread must be hand-picked.

Such treasure is within easy reach of anyone blessed with a growing season that extends into September. Saffron is a crocus and just as easy to grow as those spring harbingers that dot your garden with early cheer. But it blooms in autumn. The bulb, or corm, is hardy, but it needs a long, hot summer extending into autumn to produce the flowers you're seeking. It's worth trying, though, even if you only get flowers one year out of five; saffron crocus corms are surprisingly inexpensive, not much more than the price of regular spring bulbs.

Colour is the biggest and best of saffron's attributes. Hare Krishna devotees, denizens of Mount Olympus in Greek myth and Chinese royalty all adorned themselves with robes dyed with saffron. More practically, the blossoms also brighten the dinner plate. Just a smidgen is enough to colour rice, paella or sauces. Always be sparing with saffron, not because of its cost but because of its taste – the strong medicinal flavour is sprightly in tiny quantities but overpowering and bitter in larger amounts.

Plant saffron in its own place of honour in the herb garden, or with autumn-blooming friends such as purple asters or red salvias. It forms clumps of grassy leaves when not in bloom.

saffron rice with cardamom pods

1 Heat 4 tbsp olive oil in a large saucepan. Add 400 g basmati rice and a pinch of saffron thread about 5 mm long. Stir over medium heat until rice is translucent. Add 1 litre water and bring it to the boil.

2 Stir in 6–12 dried cardamom pods. Reduce heat to low, to keep rice at a simmer. Cover with a tight lid. Do not stir. After 15 minutes, check if water is absorbed. If not, replace lid for another 5 minutes.

3 Turn off heat and pour 200 g frozen or fresh peas atop rice. Replace the lid and leave for 10 minutes. Before serving, stir the rice with a fork. Serves 6.

planting Plant corms in well-drained, fertile soil in full sun to light shade. If you have doubts about the length of your growing season, keep in full sun.

cultivation In cold-winter areas, mulch over winter to protect from any deep-freeze spells.

harvest Use manicure scissors to snip off at its base the deep orange, three-part 'stigma' in the centre of the blossom, which at first glance looks like three leggy orange threads. Do not collect the yellow stamens around the taller, more noticeable stigma. Dry saffron threads on a sheet of paper indoors. Store in a tightly lidded glass vial.

Cucumis sativus
cucumber

Just how cool is that proverbial cucumber? Cool enough to keep your face and body moisturized, to help heal an inflammation, sunburn or a kitchen burn, and strong enough to soothe bedsores. Taken internally, this cool customer has been acclaimed for its diuretic effects in helping those with heart and kidney ailments.

Cucumbers taste best when picked before they are fully ripe, while their skin is still entirely deep green, but herbalists let the fruit ripen. Waiting until the cucumbers mature means you'll get fewer per plant, because the mission of the annual vine is to produce mature fruits capable of carrying on the next generation. When you regularly pick young cucumbers, the vine keeps trying, putting out new flowers and fruits. Enjoy it both ways: pick young ones for eating fresh or dill pickles, then let the next batch mature on the plant.

For an unlikely but appealing combination, let the vines sprawl along the ground in front of a stand of tall, tropical-looking cannas.

planting Sow seed in late spring, after soil is warm. Plant in well-drained, fertile soil, in full sun.

cultivation Grow on a trellis or use to cloak a chainlink fence. Extend mulch as vines on the ground stretch outwards.

harvest For herbal use, pick when the fruits begin to turn yellow. Use them fresh. Store any extras in the vegetable bin of your refrigerator.

a cooling facial from the garden

1 Pick one medium to large, ripe cucumber. Cool in vegetable bin overnight.

2 Peel, then finely chop the cucumber in a food processor. Gently rub the juice into your skin, then slather on the pulp.

3 Lie back and enjoy the soothing facial for 10 to 15 minutes as the juice works its magic on your skin, leaving it soft and refreshed.

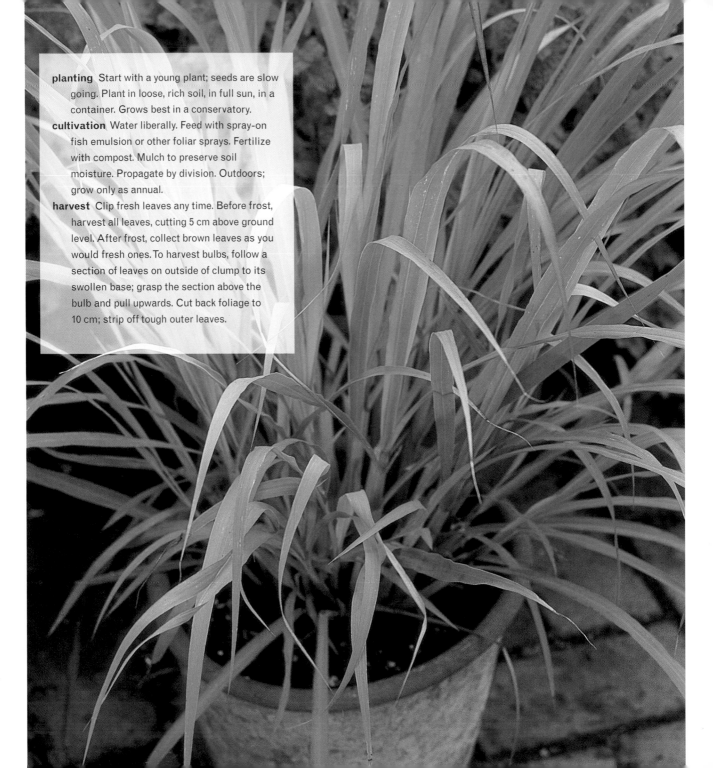

planting Start with a young plant; seeds are slow going. Plant in loose, rich soil, in full sun, in a container. Grows best in a conservatory.

cultivation Water liberally. Feed with spray-on fish emulsion or other foliar sprays. Fertilize with compost. Mulch to preserve soil moisture. Propagate by division. Outdoors; grow only as annual.

harvest Clip fresh leaves any time. Before frost, harvest all leaves, cutting 5 cm above ground level. After frost, collect brown leaves as you would fresh ones. To harvest bulbs, follow a section of leaves on outside of clump to its swollen base; grasp the section above the bulb and pull upwards. Cut back foliage to 10 cm; strip off tough outer leaves.

Cymbopogon citratus
lemongrass

A tall, lush fountain of fragrance, this tropical grass makes an unusual addition to your herb garden. In a single season, it zooms from a puny young plant in a small starter pot to a hefty clump 1 metre tall and too big to get your arms around. That kind of record speed makes it ideal for gardens in any climate; even though freezing cold will end its life, you'll be rewarded during the growing season with an abundance of foliage for tea and other delights. If you want to be sure your plant will flourish, grow it in the greenhouse or conservatory and ensure that the temperature doesn't dip too far below about 13°C. In late autumn you can dig up a winter's worth of sweetly edible lemongrass 'bulbs' for flavouring your cooking.

Fresh lemon scent is evident as soon as you brush the grassy foliage. For an authentic taste of southeast Asian cookery, use both leaves and the bulbous swellings at the base of the stems to flavour chicken, fish, vegetables, Thai spring rolls, soups and pastas. Simmer a handful of lemongrass leaves for a mild, delicious tea or use the brew as the base for a mixed herbal tea blend, adding peppermint or chamomile to remedy stomach cramps and flatulence. The mildness of this brew is especially suitable for children. Enjoy the clean, sharp scent too, by chopping the leaves into potpourri, braiding them into a wreath or scenting the bath water. Fill a handkerchief with dried lemongrass, stitch the edges closed and lay it among your linens to give them a light fragrance. Twist a few green, strappy leaves into impromptu napkin rings for alfresco dining and your friends and family will benefit from the insect-deterring power of the plant. It's a close relative of citronella, which yields the pest-repellent oil that's a popular ingredient in patio candles.

The upright, vertical habit of lemongrass provides strong contrast to its more relaxed neighbours. For a simple and beautiful combo, fill a big pot with a plant of lemongrass, red geraniums and white cascading petunias.

storing the bounty for all-winter use

A single clump of lemongrass holds the makings for a winter's worth of tasty teas and main dishes, plus the start of next year's crop. Here's how to store the generous bounty:

1 Dry or freeze fresh green leaves, packed loosely in some zip-top plastic bags.

2 Twist frost-killed brown leaves, which are still very fragrant, into a loose coil or an open braid, so any remaining moisture can dry. Hang on the kitchen wall and slice off sections as desired.

3 Gather all the bulbs except for those in the very centre of the clump. Trim the foliage back to 10 cm and store the bulbs, unbagged, in your vegetable bin.

4 Slice out remaining clump of grass and transplant into a pot to winter indoors; in mild areas, let it grow back into a full-sized clump in the garden.

snowflakes for a winter window

1 In late summer, when plants are in full bloom, cut whole flowerheads of various sizes, leaving the tiniest bit of stem.

2 Press flowerheads between pages of a phone book. Arrange the flowers carefully so that the florets are fully spread out.

3 At winter decorating time, carefully lift out the flowers, which are about to become a flurry of snowflakes on your windows. Dab a few dots of clear-drying, 'tacky' glue in the centre of each blossom and push against the inside pane of your windows or door.

Daucus carota
carrot/Queen Anne's lace

The next time you pull the common weed called Queen Anne's lace out of the soil, sniff the root. Smell familiar? You've just evicted the forerunner of the plump orange carrots in your vegetable garden. The pale, skinny root in your hand is a medicinal plant, just not as pretty or as big a mouthful as its more civilized offspring.

One of the most common wild plants of fields and roadsides, this biennial grows a ferny clump of foliage in its first year, then elongates to a 60- to 100-cm-high stem holding lacy clusters of tiny white flowers, often dotted with purple. Grow it in cottage gardens, where it will self-sow among goldenrod, coneflowers or roses.

The carrot, a relative of Queen Anne's Lace, is valued for vitamin A, noted for improved night vision. And its roots are used in herbal medicine to soothe heartburn. However, it is wise not to use for self medication.

planting Sow seeds in spring to early autumn, in a sunny site of lean to rich soil. After the first sowing, the plants will seed themselves year after year.

cultivation Control any unwanted seedlings with mulch, or by prying out the older plants with a dandelion digger.

harvest Shake ripe seeds into paper bag for sowing next year. Clip flowers any time for pressing.

Digitalis purpurea
foxglove

With its charming speckled mittens strung along the stem, foxglove in bloom looks totally harmless. Don't be fooled by appearances: this innocent-looking biennial or perennial is actually one of the most potent and dangerous herbs, definitely not suitable for home experiments. The source of the well-known drug digitalis and its extract digitoxin, it makes the heart beat like a sledgehammer. That effect is just what doctors need for some heart patients, but its too strong to play with. The plant is so toxic that a small number of highly susceptible people may suffer rashes or nausea from prolonged handling.

Foxglove is welcome in the garden for its beauty and adaptable nature. Its gentle white, rosy purple, soft yellow or pale peach are easy to fit into colour schemes and its vertical lines add order and height. Plant in groups of at least three to avoid an unnatural lollipop look.

dangerous beauty

Vanity had a high price in days of old, when the cosmetic cupboard included such beautifiers as powdered lead to whiten the complexion, deadly nightshade to dilate the pupils for languid, come-hither eyes and foxglove for the rosy cheeks and flushed bosom caused by a pounding heart and zooming blood pressure. A beautiful corpse was often the unpleasant side effect, as these poisons led to coma, stroke and death.

One of the best showy flowering plants for shade, foxglove works magic along paths in a woodland garden, where its tall spires rise like pastel candlesticks amongst hostas and bergenia. It also enjoys sun, so use it to add old-fashioned charm to a cottage garden or traditional perennial bed. For a simple, satisfying combination, plant any colour of foxglove with deep blue-purple Siberian irises and white shasta daisies, fronted with a ruff of lady's mantle. Although the deep root resents transplanting once established, it's worth gambling on moving a few pot-grown yearling plants into a large container to make a dramatic garden centrepiece. For an unusual composition, fill in around the rosettes of a peach-coloured foxglove cultivar with ruffly, deep-toned heucheras; snuggle in white and peach verbena and some creeping thyme to drape over the pot.

planting Most cultivars bloom in their second year. Sow seeds indoors in late winter or outside in spring to early summer, so they reach a good size by winter. Plant in sun to light shade. Keep soil well-drained with plenty of gravel and compost.

cultivation Many live only a few years, but self-sown progeny ensure a continual supply. Remove flowers before they seed to encourage side buds to bloom again. Leave a few pods to self-sow.

harvest Do not use medicinally. Wear gloves to cut and arrange bouquets if you have sensitive skin.

Echinacea spp.
purple coneflower

One of the great garden finds of recent decades, this easy-care perennial was almost unheard of amongst the previous generation of gardeners. Originally a wild flower, it's blessed with abundant flowers and a long period of bloom, plus an easy-going personality. Usually untroubled by pests or diseases, it splashes gardens with colour from May through frost, attracting both admiring glances and nectaring butterflies. *Echinacea purpurea* is the most popular form; the lesser-known pale coneflower (*E. pallida*) and selections with both white and purple flowers are also gaining ground.

Prized by Native Americans for treating a laundry list of ailments from snakebite to boils to open wounds, echinacea is enjoying boom times on herbal remedy counters today thanks to its reputation for minimizing allergies and boosting the immune system. Its powers, concentrated in the roots, act as what oldtimers called a 'blood purifier', speeding up healing, stimulating the immune reaction and acting as an antibiotic.

Enjoy purple coneflower in the garden as an adaptable, reliable perennial. Its rosy colour is beautiful with yellow yarrow or tansy, or with pink and purple bergamot, and its deep roots resist being overwhelmed by those aggressively spreading neighbours. The leaves stay in a tidy, gradually expanding clump, so the plant is well behaved in more formal beds too.

Because of its long bloom period, purple coneflower can ornament a bed of roses and bearded iris, then move right along to summer daylilies without pausing for breath. Ornamental grasses are natural companions from wild days that look just as good in a garden setting. Butterflies adore the nectar-rich blossoms and goldfinches will visit as the seedheads ripen.

making echinacea extract

1 Place washed fresh roots in bowl and bruise with the back of a sturdy spoon. Scrape into an enamel or glass saucepan, using about 25 g of root per 1 litre water. Bring to boil, cover and simmer.

2 After about 15 minutes, remove the saucepan from the heat, still covered, and allow the brew to steep. When it is cool, strain out all the plant parts. Store the liquid in a glass bottle in the refrigerator.

3 Drink just 1 tbsp of the decoction, three times a day, when the allergy season is approaching, or when you are feeling tired and run-down because of a cold coming on.

planting Easy from seed, or start with plants for
bloom the same year. Sow in average to
fertile, well-drained soil in full sun to part
shade. Thrives in heavy clay soil.

cultivation Unusually and delightfully care-free.
Self-sows moderately, but extra plants are
never a problem: transplant for another
welcome spot of colour.

harvest In late autumn, dig up the entire plant.
Cut off largest roots for fresh use or drying.
Replant the rest of plant; and new growth will
appear in spring.

Elettaria cardamomum
cardamom

If you're a fan of curries and other Indian foods, you know the flavour of cardamom — warm, fruity, with a hint of ginger and cinnamon. In India, it grows as a shrub, but unless you have a greenhouse, this aromatic herb will only grow as big as a large houseplant.

In cold-winter areas, cardamom won't reach flowering and fruiting stage, but you can grow it as a point of interest, planted in a large pot to bring indoors in winter. Like other jungle plants, this has large leaves, which can be up to 30 cm long. Its stems reach over 2 metres, or larger in a heated, steamy greenhouse. Surround it with bright red cannas or flowering ginger or make it the centrepiece of a shady patio, with pots of white impatiens at its feet.

Nibble a few seeds for fresh breath or to relieve flatulence, and slip the fragrant leaves among jumpers or sheets for spicy perfume.

planting Plant roots or start with a young potted plant. Grow in rich soil in shade.

cultivation Grow outdoors only in summer. Supply abundant moisture, spraying foliage as well as soaking the soil at least twice weekly. Bring indoors in autumn; a bathroom window makes a good home due to the high humidity levels.

harvest Should pods develop, pick them when plump and use fresh or dried. Drop whole pods into rice, curries and other dishes, or remove the seeds inside the pods for use whole or ground.

Ephedra spp.
desert tea, ephedra

Native Americans, cowboys, covered wagon drivers, Mormons and brothel clientele alike embraced the stimulating effects of ephedra, a native shrub of American and Asian deserts that looks nothing more than a bushy jumble of green leafless sticks. Considered a 'blood purifier', it was also used as a cure for venereal disease.

Ephedra seemed like a miracle drug to modern herbalists, too, who incorporated it into over-the-counter energy boosters. As a natural pick-me-up, it was thought both safe and non-habit-forming. It was especially popular with long-distance lorry drivers and college students. Research in the 1990s, however, showed that ephedra, and especially the Chinese species ma-huang, are too risky to fool with (see box, right).

planting Order young plants from a nursery that specializes in unusual plants or herbs. Plant under an overhang or in the conservatory. Grow desert tea in full sun, in light, fast-draining soil. Excellent in alkaline soils.

cultivation Best in dry climates. Fill a container with half sand, half soil-less potting mix.

harvest Do not use medicinally. Traditionally, branches were cut and dried for use in 'desert tea'.

Difficult to grow in areas of Britain, ephedra is most at home in low-rainfall cimates, but it can also grow in dry spots under overhangs. This is one plant you can rely upon to still be around after a lengthy hose-pipe ban! Contrast its minimalist look with leafier plants. All varieties share the bare-stemmed look – their tiny, scale-like leaves are a water-saving adaptation. Some have red or grey stems instead of green. The plants are male or female, with barely noticeable flowers, followed by small green cones on male plants and red berries on females.

Ephedra was also used for kidney ailments, to dry up sinus problems and to control fevers. Play it safe and simply admire it for its unusual form and long history as a helping herb.

delayed dangers

The amphetamine-like action of ephedra can cause a racing heart and off-the-charts high blood pressure, leading to a heart attack and stroke. Even extended use with no ill effects can't be regarded as proof that a particular user is immune to the herb's action. It can, and does, strike without warning. Several countries appear to be heading towards a ban of ma-huang, despite its thousands of years of use in Chinese herbal medicine, and tightened controls for less potent species.

Plants that can kill often do their nefarious work quickly, numbing the tongue and throwing the unfortunate user into seizures, coma or worse. Ephedra can kill outright, felling an unsuspecting user with an immediate heart attack or stroke. But its deadly action also works in sneakier ways. The elevated blood pressure caused by ephedra gradually does serious, silent damage to your heart, blood vessels and other parts of the circulatory system. Although you may not immediately notice any alarming side effects, continued use can cause irreparable harm. Ephedra is still a component of over-the-counter diet aids, but warnings and restrictions are now beginning to be attached to its use.

Eupatorium purpureum
sweet Joe Pye

Springtime wild flowers like bluebells have been popular with gardeners for decades, but many summer and autumn bloomers have only recently been invited into the garden. Perhaps that's because many later-blooming wild flowers have pushy habits, using vigorously spreading roots or myriads of self-sown seedlings to maintain their territory.

As gardeners and plant breeders get more adventurous, wild flowers of other seasons are joining their spring-blooming brethren in the garden. Amongst the best are members of the genus *Eupatorium*, including sweet Joe Pye. All are very easy to grow and bloom at a time when there's not much else going on.

Joe Pye isn't as well known as Johnny Appleseed, but he also spread the gospel of plants for human use. Dubbed 'Joe Pye' by his white New England neighbours, the American Indian medicine man allegedly cured even typhus with the wild flower that bears his name.

Known also as king or queen of the meadow, this is one of the tallest perennials, ranging from 1 to 2 metres high. Even before it comes into its late-season glory, Joe Pye is a strong presence, due to its eye-catching foliage and stout, upright stems. Its leaves form whorls at intervals around the stem, like a series of widely spaced, stiff petticoats. In late summer through to autumn, clouds of misty mauve flowers open into huge puffs, beloved by nectar-seeking insects.

A few nearly lookalike species share similar attributes and whatever type was handy served herbalists treating kidney and urinary problems, as well as general aches and pains. Research shows use may cause kidney and liver damage, so grow sweet Joe Pye as ornament only.

Use it as the centrepiece of your herb garden or plant it near water, where it often grows in the wild. In perennial beds, partner the tall species with late-blooming sunflowers or surround the shorter version with asters and purple coneflowers. Try it with grasses too, with a splash of golden black-eyed Susans.

A bonus of butterflies is the pay-off for growing sweet Joe Pye. It is a magnet for many species, providing food before their autumn migration. The fluffy flowerheads are made up of thousands of tiny florets, each holding nectar, so butterflies will feed for minutes at a time, allowing you a close-up look.

planting Start with young plants for flowers the same year. Grow in wet to well-drained, average to rich soil, in full sun to part shade.

cultivation Plant where you want it to stay – the roots grow into a heavy mass, hard to pry out. May self-sow moderately. Cut back in late winter.

harvest Avoid using medicinally. Cut blossoms for bouquets any time; cut brown seedheads after seeds disperse, for winter arrangements. Press the florets for notecards and other crafts.

Eupatorium spp.
hemp agrimony, boneset, white snakeroot

For the shady herb garden, hemp agrimony (*E. cannabinium*) offers drifts of pink blossoms, perfect along a path or behind a bench, where it can freely colonize. Boneset (*E. perfoliatum*), a white-flowered species, was once used not to heal fractures, but to soothe the bone-deep pain of fever and flu. Boneset was also once employed to treat snakebites; in some pockets of the world, folks still say that if this herb and the related snakeroot are common, so are vipers.

Research indicates that eupatoriums may be injurious to health, possibly damaging the liver or kidneys. Even long ago, white snakeroot (*E. rugosum*) had a reputation as a poison: when eaten by cows and transferred to their milk, it caused the sometimes fatal 'milk sickness', purported by historians to have wiped out the best part of many settlements in America.

planting Start with young plants or grow from seed for bloom for the following year. Plant in sun to shade, in well-drained soil.

cultivation Best for gardens a little on the wild side; they tend to grow out of bounds quickly, either through rampant roots or self-sowing. Uproot misplaced plants by hand-pulling.

harvest Do not use medicinally. Cut fresh flowers for bouquets any time.

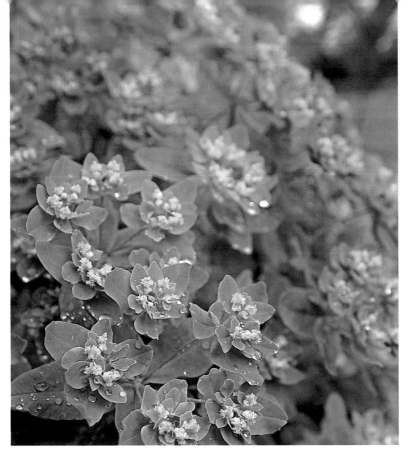

Euphorbia robbiae
spurge

The most popular euphorbia is to be found in millions of homes at Christmas time, given a place of honour for the big red flowers we know as poinsettias. Look closely at other euphorbias, and you'll see the kinship: these plants have small, yellow flowers atop a ruff of coloured bracts that look like petals. Break a stem and notice the milky juice that made them part of the herbal medicine chest.

Don't rub your fingers in that sap, though. It may cause a blistering outbreak of dermatitis. In the old days, when a thorough 'cleansing' of the system was used as a last-ditch cure, various spurges were used to empty the bowels of impurities. Think commercial laxatives times 100, add a bad case of seasickness and you have some idea of the strength of Mother Nature's 'cures'. And, as usual, the trouble centred around inexact dosage. Death was a frequent side effect of cure-by-spurge.

Treat it with respect and the various spurges will make interesting ornamental plants for the garden, as well as a conversation piece. Plant them away from paths, patios or children's play areas, to avoid accidental run-ins with the sap.

Advertisements sometimes crop up offering spurge for repelling moles. Although many species spread rapidly, burrowing animals can quickly detour around their roots. Unless you plan to cover your entire garden with spurge, its effectiveness is very questionable.

planting Start with young potted plants; most have long taproots that resent transplanting when older. Grow in well-drained lean to rich soil, in full sun to shade, depending on species.

cultivation Good for ground cover; difficult to eradicate once established. Control spread by digging or pulling up trespassers. Wear gloves and long-sleeved shirt when handling spurge. Avoid touching your gloved hand to any bare skin. Hardiness varies.

harvest Do not use for medicinal purposes. Do not cut flowers, to prevent accidental touching of the plant.

Foeniculum vulgare
fennel

Ever wonder how Roman ladies kept so slim with their great feasting and indolence? Say hello to fennel, one of the earliest known aids for dieters. The liquorice-flavoured leaves and seeds of green and red fennel and the bulbs of Florence fennel were nibbled to quiet hunger pangs of ancient Greeks at sea, Anglo-Saxons on the warpath and body-conscious women of ease.

Fennel's flavour is strongest raw; it diminishes when cooked. Sprinkle leaves in salads and on fish, add seeds to bread and sauces or chop young stems for savoury-sweet crunch in salads. Steam the bulb of Florence fennel to serve with tomato or cream sauces, or eat thin, raw strips.

Fennel is a tall, delicate beauty with feathery leaves and slender, open form. A red-leaved form is even prettier to contrast with yellow, pink or white flowers. The clusters of tiny flowers draw many insects, including some beneficials.

planting Simple to grow from seed scattered on prepared soil. Grow in full sun, in average to fertile, well-drained soil.

cultivation Self-sows well. Smother excess seedlings with mulch or pull them for salads. Perennial in most areas; grow as annual in very cold areas.

harvest To harvest the 'bulb', cut plant at soil level in autumn or when base appears sufficiently swollen. Clip leaves any time. Shake seeds into a paper bag or hang over cardboard trays until they fall out naturally. Use sprigs of foliage in herbal vinegars.

fennel and blue cheese hors d'oeuvres

1 Cut plant at base. Slice off tops; save these for other use. Working as with celery, pull off individual stems or 'ribs' of fennel from the bulb.

2 Wash fennel stems. Trim to 10 cm, leaving an open 'scoop' on one end of each piece.

3 Combine 90 g of cream cheese with 1 tbsp of blue cheese. Spread onto fennel stems, as if stuffing celery.

4 Sprinkle each piece with a few caraway seeds. Garnish with a small sprig of fennel foliage. Cover with clingfilm and store in the refrigerator until ready to serve.

To help keep a
strawberry bed
vigorous, mow using a
lawnmower with the
blade set to its highest
setting (10–12 cm) in
late summer, after the
fruiting season is
finished. Rake off any
debris and watch the
plants regrow fresh
and newly invigorated.

Fragaria vesca

wild strawberry

Picked at peak flavour, warmed by the sun, popped into the mouth – sweet, tiny wild strawberries are a precious commodity. They're nearly impossible for commercial growers to exploit on a large-scale level, so you'll need to grow your own to enjoy the experience.

Luckily, these appealing plants are simple to grow. Dedicate a raised bed or other area to them or use these neat plants with their sprinkling of simple white flowers to line a path so you can simply stoop for a taste of summer. 'Fraise du bois' or Alpine strawberry (*F. vesca* 'Alexandria') grows in tidy clumps, holding leaves upwards on long stems. It is delicious and

prized by herbalists for its calming effect on nerves (whether by the pleasure of eating or by intrinsic chemical properties is open to discussion). *F. vesca* 'Variegata', which has creamy-edged leaves, does not produce fruit.

The leaves of both types can make tea to aid digestion, diarrhoea and bellyaches. Mashed and dabbed on the face, they have a drying effect that helps clear up oily skin and skin blemishes. A strawberry facial is also said to whiten skin and lighten freckles and age spots. If you have any strawberries to spare, experiment with the crushed fruit and juice.

Of course, wild strawberries add a special touch to desserts and salads. Scatter them atop vanilla pudding or serve with a pitcher of heavy cream. Or you could lay a small nosegay of the long-stemmed clusters of berries on each plate.

planting Set plants 30 cm apart in rich, loose, well-drained soil. Fruiting is better when planted in sun.

cultivation These are prolific plants, with each parent sending out several new plantlets on runners during the season. Transplant these to another location to expand the plantings. Cover with netting to protect from the birds. Mulch well to keep the fruit clean.

harvest Pick berries when they are red and sweet. Eat fresh, dry or freeze. Clip the leaves any time for drying. Avoid using the leaves when fresh as they will still contain toxins.

Galium odoratum
sweet woodruff

Sniff a plant of sweet woodruff and you're likely to wonder what all the fuss is about. The only fragrance you will be able to discern smells vaguely green, certainly not anything that could be called sweet. Now, dry a leaf for about a week and try the sniff test again. Sweet indeed, with the perfumes of vanilla and new-mown hay.

Sweet woodruff spreads rapidly into a dense ground cover of deep green foliage, highlighted by sprays of starry white flowers in spring. It sulks in sun but spreads happily in shade, even in difficult areas where a heavy network of tree roots competes for moisture and nutrients. Plant it as a ground cover, accented with hostas and ferns. Fill in that forgotten deeply shaded strip beside the garage with this agreeable plant and before you know it you'll be considering that former wasteland as a new garden.

German May wine is traditionally flavoured by dried, sweet woodruff, a practice dating back to the Middle Ages. After quaffing a bowl of wine, participants at May Day feasts may have slept on mattresses containing sweet woodruff – an excellent camouflage for body odours. Indeed, the sweet scent of woodruff masked a multitude of unpleasant smells: it was used to make stale rooms bearable, cover up sewage odours and even mask the scent of a body laid out for burial.

In modern homes, sweet woodruff lends its pleasant fragrance to dried arrangements and potpourris. Use handfuls of dried foliage in herbal wreaths or to fill a wide, shallow bowl for your hall. Show off the interesting whorled leaves, arranged in frills around the bare stem, by pressing several sprigs and arranging them in a frame as a botanical wall hanging.

planting Start with young plants; seed can be quite difficult to germinate. Plant in well-drained soil, in part to full shade.

cultivation Plants multiply fast by sending out running roots, from which new stems of greenery arise. Be sure to choose a location where woodruff can stay; eradicating it is painstaking work, because every small, overlooked bit of the brittle roots will regrow as a new plant.

harvest You can cut the stems of foliage at any time, clipping them close to the ground with scissors. Dry before use.

a sweet scent to dream on

Perfume your pillow with the old-fashioned aroma of new-mown hay by tucking a few sprigs of dried, sweet woodruff among the pillowcases in your linen cupboard. For a stronger scent, refreshed every time you move your head, slip a sprig of dried greenery directly inside your pillowcase. Arrange it near the top of the pillow, to avoid being disturbed like the princess and the pea. As you move your head during sleep, the pressure of the cloth against the foliage will release a light waft of perfume.

Glechoma hederacea
ground ivy, gill-over-the-ground

Chances are you may already be playing host to ground ivy. It's a common weed in many areas of Britain and often slips on the roots of plants such as daylilies, irises or other frequently swapped plants from friends or neighbours – unintentionally of course!

With its small, scalloped-edge leaves and dainty blue flowers, plus a solid reputation as a remedy for nasal congestion, this perennial herb can be a charmer at first. But it is highly invasive and nearly impossible to un-invite once rooted. If you already have it, celebrate its strengths and forgive its Napoleonic tendencies. After all, aren't we always looking for a pretty, indestructible ground cover that will thrive in even the worst soil? If you can, restrict its spread to beneath shrubs or among lawngrass. Weed it out when it crops up among plants of weaker constitutions, such as creeping thymes, which could be swallowed in one gulp.

planting If you have it, learn to live with it. If you don't, do not bring it into your garden.
cultivation Control by hand-weeding, making sure to remove every bit of the rooting stems. Dispose of unwanted plants on bonfire, not the compost pile.
harvest Whirl half a cup of water and a handful of fresh foliage and stems, gathered any time, in a blender or juicer to make juice. Take 1 tsp, two or three times a day, to relieve congestion.

Hamamelis virginiana
witch hazel

Witch hazel is an unusual character: it blooms in very early spring, long before most flowers wake up. In snowy areas, the incongruity of witch hazel is a complete delight when its flurry of golden flowers is topped with an icing of snow.

A common ingredient in astringents and in rubbing alcohol, witch hazel has a sharp, medicinal smell. It has been used as a gargle, to heal mouth inflammation and as a poultice for tired or inflamed eyes, as well as for skin rashes, insect bites and poison ivy. Commercial extract is used in aftershave preparations, sunburn lotions and cosmetics. Because the active properties are found in the bark of this woody shrub and require special methods to extract the volatile oils, it is difficult to gather more than a very small quantity at home. Buy witch hazel water at chemists and plant the shrub as an item of interest rather than a source.

You can also try your luck at another old-time use of witch hazel, still employed by gifted 'dowsers' and other countryfolk all around the world. The forked branches are highly flexible, which makes them ideal for use as divining rods. In the hands of a 'water dowser', the forked stick is held before the body, with the single end of the branch pointing outwards. When the dowser walks over a source of water, the witch hazel jerks downwards, pointing to the spot where a new well should be dug. Forty-niners in the California goldrush transferred this skill to seeking out underground lodes of the gleaming metal; whether or not witch hazel was their instrument of choice is not recorded.

Witch hazel may not lead you to the mother lode, but it is definitely a garden treasure. Besides its welcome, offbeat flowers, this woody shrub or small tree has a graceful form that is most evident in winter after the leaves drop. Other witch hazel species are equally worthy of a home in your garden. Try the Chinese variety *H. mollis* or other modern hybrids, the offspring of a marriage between Chinese and Western forms. These tend to have showier flowers, as well as a wider colour range. Underplant witch hazel with snowdrops, early crocus and other spring bulbs plus a few clumps of bluebells, which will come into bloom just as the tender new leaves of the witch hazel begin to appear.

planting Plant a young shrub in average to fertile, well-drained soil. Witch hazel grows best in shade, which mimics its natural woodland habitat, but it will also flourish in sun.

cultivation Water well for the first two years if rainfall is scarce. Propagate by layering. Remove suckers at ground level to keep a single trunk; hybrids may be grafted onto the root of a different species from which suckers are growing.

harvest Collect branches any time. Clip stems of flowers for bouquets whenever they are in bloom.

soothe tired eyes

1 Clip off a branch of witch hazel at least 15 cm long using secateurs. Strip off the bark, using a paring knife. Add 2 tbsp bark to 500 ml water in a glass or enamel saucepan.

2 Cover and boil for about 10 minutes. Remove from the heat and steep, covered, for about 15 minutes. Strain out all the plant parts. Allow the liquid to cool.

3 Moisten cotton balls in the witch hazel decoction. Put your head back (or lie down) and apply to your closed eyelids for between 5 to 10 minutes.

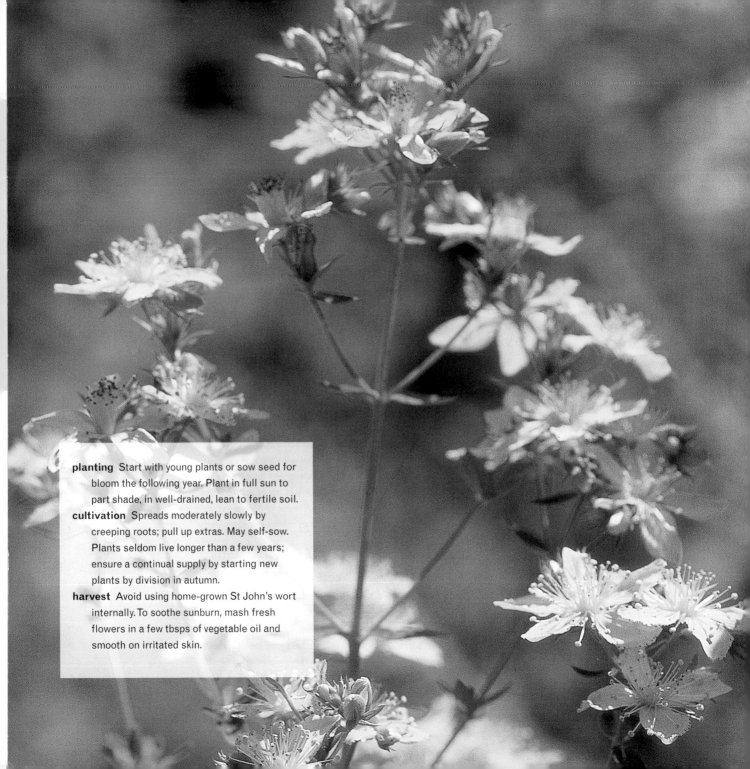

planting Start with young plants or sow seed for bloom the following year. Plant in full sun to part shade, in well-drained, lean to fertile soil.

cultivation Spreads moderately slowly by creeping roots; pull up extras. May self-sow. Plants seldom live longer than a few years; ensure a continual supply by starting new plants by division in autumn.

harvest Avoid using home-grown St John's wort internally. To soothe sunburn, mash fresh flowers in a few tbsps of vegetable oil and smooth on irritated skin.

Hypericum spp.
St John's wort

Until the last decade, this was an unassuming yellow-flowered perennial, a common weed of fields, roadsides and wasteland. Its name was known only to wild flower enthusiasts and many of them scorned it.

Still rarely recognized along the highways and byways, its name is now familiar to millions of people throughout the world. That's because the all-too-common malady of modern life, depression, can be greatly alleviated by the action of this humble weed.

As herbal practitioners began advertising the herb as a cure for mild depression, St John's wort was suddenly a star in the non-prescription department of every herb shop and chemist. Instead of paying high prices for popular prescription drugs, like Prozac, people turned in droves to the inexpensive, plant-based relief of this natural cure. First documented in European studies, St John's wort is so effective at lifting the spirits and restoring a sense of well-being that it holds a solid position among the top ten commercially made herbal products. (Photosensitivity is a common side effect: during treatment, the skin may become hypersensitive to sunlight, resulting in inflammation and dermatitis.)

To modern fans, St John's wort seems like a miracle. To ancient aficionados, the plant was no less magical: they used it to banish evil spirits and to predict the day of death. The herb gets its name from John the Baptist, for whom the plant was said to 'bleed' on the anniversary of the saint's beheading. You can try the memorial effect yourself – pinch a yellow petal and it will turn blood red. A reddish oil may also occasionally seep from the porelike glands near the edges of the leaves, especially when you crush the foliage.

St John's wort ('wort' is an old English word meaning 'plant') blooms in mid- to late summer. Place a clump near a path in the herb garden so that you can show off its colour-changing trick and inhale the sharp, piney smell of its foliage. Let it mingle with ornamental grasses, whose golden winter colour will be a warm backdrop for the dark seedheads of St John's wort.

very important – don't try this at home

The active compounds of herbs are not always the same. Depending on the soil, the climate, the time of day, the maturity of the plant when it is picked and a host of other variables, the volatile oils, acids, proteins and other elements can veer from mild to potent. That's why experimenting with medicinal herbs can be a risky proposition. Brain chemistry especially is a delicate balance; don't take chances with home-grown. If you are interested in trying the effects of St John's wort, turn to commercial products that guarantee reliable proportions of ingredients based on chemical analysis.

Hyssopus officinalis
hyssop

The pungent aroma of hyssop is a complex mix of flavours: liquorice and mint with a bitter tang. To some noses, the plant smells like mothballs or Vicks salve. In cooking, the flavour stands up to robust meats and savoury stews and sauces. A few snippets of its flowers or fine leaves add piquancy to salads and even fruit pies.

With such a strong medicinal scent, hyssop was a natural for home doctoring. Its foliage is known to host penicillin mould, and the oil in the plant also has antibiotic properties. Sixteenth-century herbalist John Parkinson noted that, 'A decoction thereof taketh away the itching and tingling of the head, and vermin also breeding therein'. Once used for treating rheumatism, whooping cough and even leprosy, hyssop oil is no longer recommended for medicinal use either internally or externally because it causes muscle spasms and even epileptic seizures. For irregular culinary use, however, small amounts of foliage or flowers, fresh or dried, are deemed safe.

Hyssop flowers are a beautiful rich blue and are produced for months. Elevate a container of hyssop on an overturned clay pot as the centrepiece of a bed of herbs, where you will get a good view of the many bees, butterflies and beneficial hoverflies attracted to the abundant flowers. In ornamental beds and borders, mix its fine texture with plants with larger leaves and simpler flowers. For an appealing trio, plant hyssop with white petunias and yellow daylilies.

planting Sow seeds or start with young plants. Grows well in full sun to light shade, in well-drained soil. Thrives in sandy and rocky soils.

cultivation A trouble-free perennial, excellent for knot gardens or as a low hedge. Stems become woody with age. Propagate by cuttings of flexible green stems. Also self-sows moderately. Cut back in late winter, removing old heads to keep it compact.

harvest Collect flowers and new leaves any time, to eat fresh or to dry for potpourri, cookery or flavouring tea.

Inula helenium
elecampane, horseheal

Elecampane has a reputation for soothing the hacking cough of bronchitis, as well as asthma flare-ups and other breathing difficulties. You can try its effectiveness yourself by steeping a teaspoon of dried, crushed root in 500 ml of water and sipping it as a tea. Add honey to make it palatable; the roots are bitter. The name 'scabwort' was also bestowed on this herb because of its healing effects on scabies, acne, cold sores and other skin outbreaks.

Big, tough and reliable, this herb holds a bouquet of fringed yellow daisies during the summer months. The stout leaves, with velvety grey undersides, may reach 60 cm long at the base of the plant. This rugged perennial is best at the back of the border or in a meadow garden, where it can show off its 1- to 3-metre height with other tall companions, such as mauve sweet Joe Pye, coneflowers and asters.

planting Sow seed or start with young plants for flowers the first year and a root harvest the second. Plant in full sun to light shade, in fertile soil.
cultivation Choose a permanent site; removal needs persistence as new plants grow from tiny pieces of root. Grows well in clay soil, but to ease digging, lighten heavy soils with compost before planting. Mulch to keep moist. Propagate by slicing plantlets off base of parent or transplanting sections of root.
harvest Dig roots in late autumn, after plant is at least two years old. Dry and grind in a food processor.

Ipomoea spp.
morning glories

Only early risers get to fully appreciate the glorious silken-petalled flowers of these annual or perennial vines, which open with the sun and fade by noon. A fresh crop of blooms is produced every day, from summer to autumn.

The seeds of the common morning glory (*I. purpurea*) were popular for a brief moment during the heyday of hippies because of their alleged hallucinogenic properties. Any such effect was due to toxins that were far too dangerous for experimentation and morning glories quickly fell out of favour as a self-administered herb. Grow the beautiful flowers on a trellis to add height to your garden and enjoy them, perhaps, as a nostalgic reminder of a more foolish youth.

Morning glory can be used to great effect by combining it with other twinery herbs like green or golden leaved hop plants (*Humulus lupus* 'Aureus'). Grown with climbing beans they attract insects to help pollinate the bean flowers and therefore help to produce a bumper crop.

planting Soak seeds overnight to hasten germination. Plant directly in garden, in full sun, in well-drained, lean to fertile soil; or grow in pots. Keep soil well-moistened until seeds sprout, then water weekly if rain is scarce.

cultivation Supply strings or a trellis for the vines to climb. Some species self-sow.

harvest Do not use medicinally. The thin-petalled flowers press beautifully for decorating gifts or using on notecards.

Laurus nobilis
sweet bay, bay laurel

Nobility is built into the Latin name of the bay tree, an evergreen from Mediterranean regions with a long and colourful history. A wreath or garland of the shining leaves signified victory with grace and honour and immediately put the wearer in high regard. The original Olympic champions were draped with bay laurel and brave generals and inspired poets proudly wore the wreath. Of course, so did Emperor Nero and other infamous corrupt characters, who defamed the noble image of the laurel wreath.

Bay was also esteemed as powerful protection from all kinds of bad things. It was credited with warding off the plague, as well as devils and witches, who were supposed to quickly flee from the power of a bay tree. Delphic priestesses consumed mass quantities of leaves before making mysterious pronouncements about the future in a hypnotic trance. In Greek myth, an unwilling female target of Apollo's affections took the form of a bay tree to escape the lusty god's advances. If Greek gods and evil spirits aren't troubling you, you may still find bay a comfort during storms. According to the old herbalists, this noble evergreen has the power to protect anyone near it from violent acts of nature.

Our use of bay laurel today has switched from the ceremonial to the stewpot. Its aromatic leaves add personality to mild cream soups and rice dishes and they intensify the flavour of tomato sauces and marinades. Use the leaves fresh or dried and rub them before dropping them into the pot. Keep count of the leaves you use so that you can be certain to remove them before serving your food. The pointy leaf would be a nasty surprise for diners!

Bay grows well in most areas of the Midlands and southern England. Even in unusually severe winters when growth is cut back, it will regenerate from the roots. In the North, on the other hand, bay may prove tender and be killed by freezing cold. However, it thrives in container culture. Enjoy your potted bay as a patio plant in the summer and when frost nears, move it indoors for the cold season.

planting Buy a young potted plant. Grow in full sun to partial shade, in rich, well-drained soil. Plant in a container in cold areas.

cultivation In containers, bay eventually grows to about 1.5 metres tall. It can reach 12 metres in-ground in the warmest areas of the South, but elsewhere grows to 3–5 metres. Cuttings of tender green stems are difficult to root; use rooting hormone and be patient. It may take over 6 months.

harvest Clip off leaves any time for fresh use or drying. Leaves curl as they dry; to keep them flat, hold them in place with corrugated cardboard. Cut back branches as desired to shape the plant; bay is often pruned into a formal-looking 'standard', with all lower branches removed to expose the bare trunk and the top shaped into a rounded head.

Lavandula spp.
lavenders

Everyone loves lavender – it smells sublime, it looks beautiful, it's easy to grow and its very name evokes the romance of the Victorian era. Perfume is one of the most ancient of lavender's uses: the herb was dropped into the bathwater of ancient Rome, slipped into the bosom of a gown to delight any nose that came near and strewn in sickrooms to freshen the air. Old-time smelling salts, sniffed by women who felt faint, combined the sweet scent of lavender oil with the sharp odour of ammonia. Lavender was also used as a moth repellent, a toothache remedy, 'to comfort and dry up the moisture of a cold braine', and to ease flatulence or nausea.

Most preparations use oil distilled from blooms at their height. In full flower, the hills of France's lavender-growing countryside and the fields of Norfolk glow in misty blue-purple, as they await harvesting for the perfume industry.

A fondness for lavender can be the start of a lifelong collection: herb catalogues simply offer so many species, cultivars and hybrids. English lavenders (*L. angustifolia*), such as 'Munstead', 'Hidcote' and dozens more, usually have darker flowers and bloom earlier than other types. *Lavandula* x *intermedia* varieties are hybrids with taller plants and larger flower spikes. Spanish or French lavenders (*L. stoechas*) have unusual stocky heads, topped by a tuft of pale to deep purple. Some of these will grow from seed, flowering by late summer.

Use fragrant lavenders with abandon throughout the garden. They look wonderful edging a brick walkway, underplanting roses, or flanking a door with potted plants. Planting them next to a garden bench will allow you to watch the butterflies and other nectar-seekers that come flocking when it blooms.

making a lavender bell

Make lavender your signature scent by tucking a lavender wand among your special stationery or in a box of all-purpose envelopes. To refresh the fragrance, just roll the beribboned head of the wand between your palms.

1 Cut about 6 to 9 fresh flowering stems of lavender, any variety, with a length of bare stem beneath the flowers.

2 Holding the bunch at the base of the flowers, bend the bare stems backwards, one by one, over the flowers.

3 Arrange the bent stems so that they form a cage, with the bent bare stems on the outside and the flowers in the middle.

4 Beginning at the bend in the stems, which will be the top of the wand, weave a 3-mm-wide satin ribbon under and over each bare stem, continuing around the entire bundle. Use a needle to coax the ribbon into place if necessary. Lay the loose end of the ribbon along the flower spike; it will be covered as you finish wrapping.

5 Repeat, making as many rows as needed to cover the flowerheads.

6 When your weaving reaches the bottom of the flower spike, knot the ribbon around the stems and tie it with a dainty bow. The bundle of bare stems that extend from the weaving are the handle of your bell.

planting Slow from seed, except for some *L. stoechas*; buy young plants instead. Grow in well-drained fertile soil in full sun.

cultivation In spring, trim back established plants to keep them shapely and compact. Do not cut as far back as woody stems; they will not regrow. Cut back after flowering, removing seed stalks. Propagate from cuttings of flexible young stems in spring.

harvest Trim off flower spikes soon after opening; dry and use whole or strip flowers for potpourri and sachets. Cut foliage from spring through late summer for drying.

planting Sow seed or set young plants in full sun
to shade, in poor to fertile, well-drained soil.
cultivation Evergreen basal leaves persist in
winter, adding colour to the garden. Spreads
by creeping roots and by self-sowing; hoe off
unwanted seedlings.
harvest Do not use medicinally. Avoid contact
with bare skin.

Leonurus cardiaca
motherwort

A common plant of roadsides and woods' edges in most areas of Britain, motherwort looks something like a delphinium plant out of bloom. At flowering time, however, the difference is distinct: instead of delphinium's tall spire of beautiful blue flowers, motherwort bears tiny, pale purple or white flowers tucked against the stem at the upper leaves.

Although its name leads us to believe the herb was useful for childbirth, this mother's helper was named for easing the symptoms of the menopause. An infusion of 1 teaspoon leaves steeped in 125 ml of water was swallowed in a dosage of 'one mouthful' per day to alleviate hot flushes, as well as to reduce the pains of arthritis, sciatica and neuralgia. The word *cardiaca* in the herb's botanical name alludes to its long-ago use as a heart stimulant, a good reason to grow the plant only as a curiosity in the modern herb garden.

Use motherwort as a background plant, where its 1-metre height and toothed leaves can serve as a cool green backdrop for silvery herbs or bright-flowered plants. Brushing bare skin against the foliage may result in dermatitis in some susceptible individuals; wear long sleeves and gloves when handling the plant, to be on the safe side. Its flowers are highly attractive to bees, another good reason to keep the plant away from the path of traffic.

Liatris spicata
gay feather, blazing star

Gay feather is a plant that has only recently come to the attention of gardeners. Its bright purple-pink fuzzy spikes aren't as familiar yet as the rosy daisies of coneflowers, but they are quickly gaining ground, thanks to their hardiness, adaptability and long-lasting flowers. Butterfly enthusiasts quickly learned that it works like a magnet for the stunning painted ladies and peacocks of summer.

Gay feather was greatly prized by early herbal practitioners because the tuberous roots of this plant were used as an attempted cure for venereal diseases.

Modern drugs have made gay feather treatments obsolete, but the flowers are still more than welcome for their bright dash of summer colour. The most commonly grown species, *L. spicata*, is a tall, showy plant, also called blazing star for its bright, cheerful purple spikes. Plant it with purple coneflowers and goldenrod for vivid summer colour.

----

planting Most economical from bulbs, planted in spring or autumn. Or buy young potted plants. Set in full sun, in fertile, well-drained soil.

cultivation Drought tolerant. Long bloom period. Propagate by digging up clump in early spring and separating bulbs.

harvest Not recommended for medicinal use. Cut fresh flowers any time for long-lasting bouquets.

sore throat or snakebite

In America, gay feather is one of many herbs that were used for a lot of unrelated ailments. Settlers with a sore throat could gargle with the same decoction they swallowed to treat more serious symptoms of the private parts. The scaly variety (*L. squarrosa*) served as first aid for rattlesnake bites; after the venom was sucked out of the wound, the root was applied to finish drawing out the poison.

Linum spp.
flax

One of the oldest crops in cultivation, flax provided the wrappings for Egyptian mummies, the sails for Roman ships and the oil for Italian master painters. The burial shroud of Turin, whose provenance is still in dispute, is made of linen produced from flax. So are the translucent pages of old Bibles, as well as early cigarette papers and modern high-quality stationery.

The flax plant has delicacy written all over it, from its ethereal, sky-blue blossoms that tremble with every slight shift of breeze, to its thin, fine stems and tiny needle-like leaves. Behind this graceful personality, though, is one tough customer. The tissue-thin linen blouses and soft, thick linen trousers we know today are a far cry from hopsacking and linsey-woolsey, which were woven from home-grown flax and prepared by hand. New clothes were more torture than delight in those days: they required a long breaking-in period before they stopped chafing.

weightloss wonder or diet dud?

Flax seeds enjoyed a boomlet of popularity in recent years as a much-touted aid to losing weight. Most customers didn't come back for a refill, however, because the way in which the pounds were shed had more to do with oil's laxative properties than with some magical fat-melting ingredient. Once used as a constipation cure to rid the bowels of the 'poisons' that supposedly caused various illnesses, flax seeds swell up in the intestines as they absorb water. Before long, the innocent user is indeed losing ounces and pounds, but not in the hoped-for manner.

Oil-rich flax seeds fed oxen, cattle and humans alike for thousands of years. Today, commercially grown seeds of annual flax (*L. usitatissimum*) are used for linseed oil, and in animal feeds and birdseed mixes – they're a favourite of finches.

To the herbalist, flax was indispensable. A tea made from the gluey crushed seeds cured coughs and colds, and supposedly halted urinary infections. Unfortunately, an overdose might also cause staggering, gasping for breath and eventual paralysis due to toxic compounds in them. A safer treatment is to grind and boil the seeds for a poultice for burns and skin sores.

Plant three or more clumps together in the herb garden or in flowerbeds, to increase the impact of their willowy stems and dainty flowers. The blossoms fade by late morning, but a new batch of blue will open the next day. The delicate colour and texture is beautiful with bold flowers, such as daisies, poppies or bearded iris.

planting Easy from seed or buy young plants. Grow in full sun, in well-drained, average to rich soil.
cultivation Self-sows moderately. Learn to recognize seedlings so you may transplant them.
harvest Gather only fully ripe seeds; unripe seeds are high in toxins. Clip seedheads and shake the shiny brown seeds into a tray to dry for a week or so. More than 300 kg of fibre can be reaped from a single acre of the plants, which are pulled up and soaked for weeks to rot the stems off the threads.

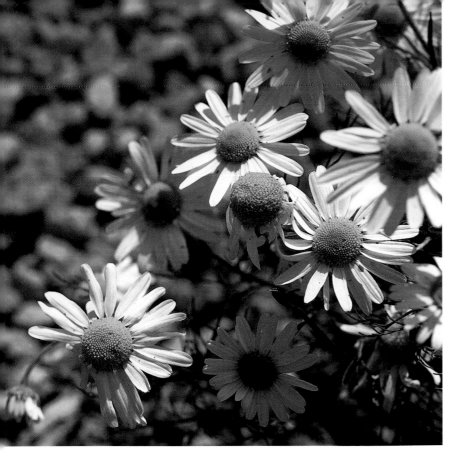

Matricaria recutita
German chamomile

You'll want to dedicate a patch of your herb garden to German chamomile so that you have bountiful makings for tea and potpourri within easy gathering reach. But do allow the plants to self-sow and snuggle into unexpected corners too. Scatter chamomile seeds beneath roses for a charming lace collar all summer long or grow a mixed bed of edible flowers by sprinkling seeds of chamomile, borage and calendula in the same patch of prepared soil.

Both German chamomile and perennial chamomile (*Chamaemelum nobile*, see pages 100–101) are well known as calming herbs and that reputation includes muscle tightness as well as nervous anxiety. Brew the flowers into a strong tea and add to a hot bath for a relaxing soak. The blossoms have antiseptic properties; gargle with cold tea to soothe mouth ulcers or sore throat. To make blonde hair shine, steep 500 ml of blossoms in 2 litres of boiling water for 30 minutes; strain, cool and pour slowly over hair. If you are allergic to pollen, you may experience symptoms from such treatments.

planting Scatter seed in autumn or spring on prepared soil. Grow in full sun, in well-drained soil.
cultivation Make successive sowings every few weeks for a continual supply of this annual.
harvest Clip off flowers when fully open, for fresh use or drying. Store in tightly sealed glass jars.

grow a gift of sleepytime tea

The light apple scent, warm liquid and calming action of the herb make chamomile tea the ideal before-bed beverage. The dried blossoms look great packed loosely into a sealed glass jar. Add a pretty label with the recipe: Put 1 to 2 tsp chamomile flowerheads in a tea ball in a cup. Fill with boiling water. Steep for a few minutes, then remove the tea ball and add honey to taste.

Melissa officinalis
lemon balm

The clean, fresh lemon scent of this perennial is wonderful in teas and a pleasure to sniff as you stroll the garden. But too much of a good thing can quickly become the case, as it spreads by creeping roots and has a habit of self-sowing to the point of weediness. Strays are easy to uproot or smother with mulch when very young, though, so don't let the plant's profligacy deter you from trying it. The flowers are also manna to bees.

Lemon is a popular scent in aromatherapy, reputed to clear the mind, sharpen memory and relieve headaches and depression. Try it yourself by bruising and inhaling the aroma of a leafy stem. Lemon balm was also said to cure the effects of mad dog bites, prevent baldness and even restore a 'crooked neck'.

Grow it in its own raised bed. Forms with golden or variegated foliage are also available, which do not spread so prolifically.

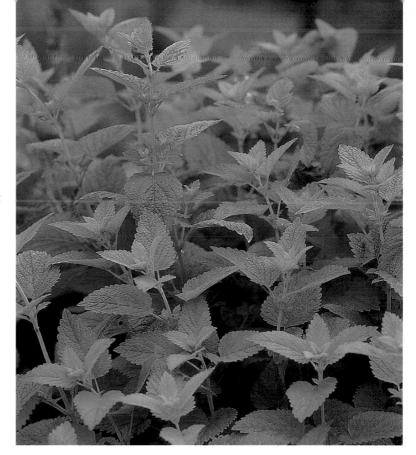

custom tea blends

Lemon balm produces so much foliage that you can easily harvest a season's supply from a single plant with three successive cuttings. Dried leaves make an excellent, mild lemony base for hot or iced teas. Combine it with one or more of the following to create your own special tea blends:

anise seeds, basil, bergamot, chamomile, cardamom pod, fennel seeds, hibiscus petals, peppermint, rose hips

planting Sow seed or start with young plants. Grow in full sun to shade, in well-drained soil. Plants may become floppy in shade; cut back as needed to keep them compact.

cultivation Slow down self-sowing by cutting plant halfway back after flowering, before seeds form. Uproot stragglers by hand.

harvest Fresh leaves make the most flavourful tea. Gather before flowers open. For large quantities, cut entire plant at ground level. Air dry on screens for winter use. Add stronger herbs for more flavour.

Mentha x piperita
peppermint

The mints are a large family of plants that have been treasured for millennia for their medicinal properties. Several species carry scents so familiar we can identify them with our eyes closed. The most familiar are peppermint and spearmint (see page 142). Rub a leaf and you'll immediately recognize the pungent aroma of menthol: the scent of mint chewing gum, breath-freshening after-dinner mints and many other delicious foods and helpful medicines.

Peppermint tea is one of the best remedies for an upset stomach. Chewing a few fresh leaves also relieves mild indigestion or flatulence. The herb is also said to relieve insomnia and it may help soothe migraines. Chopped and tied in muslin, the fresh leaves can be dropped into the bath to quiet the itch of winter-dry skin.

For a refresher of a different sort, try a homemade mint julep to celebrate summer. Use the back of a spoon to crush 6 to 10 fresh peppermint leaves against the side of a bowl. Add 1 jigger of bourbon and 1 tablespoon quick-dissolving sugar; stir well. Fill serving glass with crushed ice; strain bourbon/mint mixture into the ice. Churn up and down with a metal spoon until thoroughly mixed. Top off with more crushed ice, top with a fresh sprig and add a straw for sipping. Alternatively, try fresh mint and lemon balm tea as it makes a delicious, cooling summer drink.

planting Mints hybridize readily, so start with young plants that come from a reliable source and sniff-test them first. Plant in well-drained to moist soil, in full sun to shade.

cultivation Mint can spread rampantly (see page 142 for control suggestions). If the patch is large, mow it with the blade set at its highest setting in early summer for a fresh flush of compact growth. Hand-pull carefully, any bits of underground stems will quickly sprout anew.

harvest Collect foliage any time for use fresh or dried. To harvest large amounts, clip off plants at ground level before flowering time.

Mentha pulegium
pennyroyal

Ground-hugging pennyroyal has a different look from most common mints. Its neat, shining leaves form a thick carpet as the plant expands, topped by stems of lavender-blue flowers in late summer. It's easier to keep in bounds than the taller, more aggressive mints; try it as an underplanting for roses, where its strong scent may help repel insect pests. The thick green carpet is also attractive when it creeps amongst rocks or stepping stones.

Sometimes known as English pennyroyal, this herb smells somewhat like peppermint, with a hotter, spicier undertone. Upright pennyroyal shares the signature aroma, but is different in that it has upright, branching flowers.

Neither is edible. In fact, the oil in pennyroyal is a deadly toxin that can destroy the kidneys when taken internally. The herb was occasionally administered to induce abortion but often proved deadly to the mother as well as the baby. Keep these plants out of your mint patch, where they may be mistakenly picked for internal use, and away from other edible plants.

Pennyroyal does have its useful side. Its odour repels insects, especially ants. If ants cover your patio, plant pennyroyal around its edges to help deter them. Try rubbing pennyroyal on doorsteps and windowsills if ants invade the house.

planting Buy young plants; pennyroyal is slow to start from seed. Best in well-drained soil, in partial sun.
cultivation Water regularly if rains are scarce. Propagate by division.
harvest Do not use internally. Pick fresh leaves any time to crush against insect stings or bites.

deodorize your fingertips

Preparing fish, chopping onions, peeling garlic or smoking cigarettes can leave your fingers with a telltale aroma. To magically remove unpleasant odours from your fingers, rub a leaf of a strong-smelling mint between them until the odour is gone. Pennyroyal, peppermint and spearmint are particularly fast-acting deodorants. If you use pennyroyal, be sure to wash your hands with soap and water afterwards.

Mentha spicata
spearmint

keeping mints in check

Mints are notorious for rampant spreading. To keep your herb garden from being swallowed alive, try these tricks:

1 Give mints an area where they can freely roam, perhaps a hard-to-mow slope or the strip of soil by sheds or pathways.

2 For a small mint patch, cut out the bottom of a plastic bucket and bury it so the top rim extends 8 cm above ground. Plant mint inside.

3 Paint a child's stiff plastic swimming pool deep green-black. Fill two-thirds deep with soil and plant inside.

4 Grow mints in water: a few stems in a big jar of water will root quickly and grow for months.

Like many mints, this creeping favourite is easily hybridized and there is a huge range of varieties to choose from. Spearmint is also often to be found in the wild, especially along streams where it spreads into thick, fragrant beds.

The scent is instantly recognizable to anyone who has ever unwrapped a stick of spearmint-flavoured chewing gum. In herbal lore, its uses are similar to those for peppermint: it works as a stomach soother, to ease indigestion, nausea and heartburn. Simmer a handful of fresh, bruised leaves for tea or nibble on the greenery. It's also a great remedy for bad breath.

Less intense than peppermint, this is a favourite in cooking. It's traditionally served with spring lamb and can also be used for cold mint juleps, and even jam; add some fresh leafy stems to a mild apple jam in the last minutes of cooking.

planting Start with young plants from a reputable source; the strength of scent in seed-grown plants varies widely. Plant in sun to shade, wet to dry soil.
cultivation Controlling the plants is the trickiest part. Uproot strays ruthlessly.
harvest Gather foliage any time. For large amounts to dry, cut them at ground level before flowering time.

Monarda spp.
bergamot, beebalm

Want butterflies in your garden? Plant bright red bergamot and they will come. Bees and butterflies simply can't resist the nectar-filled flowerheads. Other colours of bergamot also satisfy their sweet tooth, but red is key to tempting them to your garden for the first time.

Bergamot has odd-looking flowers, but if you take a close look, you'll see why they're perfect for butterflies. Each shaggy head is actually a cluster of many tubular flowers, each facing outwards so that it is perfectly positioned for insects. The foliage below the flowers is what gives this herb its name: it has a light, citrusy scent like that of bergamot oranges.

A member of the mint family, as you can tell from the square stems, bergamot makes delicious tea that was first brewed by Oswego Indians in America. It can quiet an upset stomach and relieve flatulence and nausea. Oswego tea was also quaffed to soothe a cough or sore throat and to relieve menstrual cramps.

Originally a North American native, bergamot became a popular garden and tisane plant in Europe after settlers sent back seed. There are several species, all of which can be used for making tea. *Monarda didyma* blooms red in the wild, although plant breeders have developed a further range of colours from white to purple; it is often found near water or in shady woods, although it thrives in sunny gardens too. Mauve *M. fistulosa* is native to dry open fields where it blooms in late summer with goldenrod and asters. All bergamots are well suited to meadow gardens, where they can spread at will, or to flowerbeds, where they require a firm hand to keep in bounds. Partner bergamot with purple coneflowers, shasta daisies and yarrow, or let it mingle with daylilies in shades of pink and pale yellow. Bergamot flowers are edible; pull them apart and toss in salads, or dry them for long-lasting colour in potpourri. Chop young leaves and add to sliced strawberries or melon for a hint of orange flavour.

planting Start with young plants; slow to start from seed; modern colours do not come true from seed. Plant *M. didyma* in full sun to shade, in average to wet soil. Plant *M. fistulosa* in sun, in dry to average-moisture soil.

cultivation Bergamot is a mint and it spreads fast by underground stems. Hand-pull strays to keep in bounds. Propagate by division.

harvest Cut foliage any time for use fresh or dried; for large amounts, cut entire plant at base before flowering time. Cut flowers soon after opening for bouquets, for fresh culinary use or for dried arrangements and potpourri.

homegrown acne treatment

To dry up pimples, boils and other skin outbreaks, herbalists turned to wild bergamot (*M. fistulosa*). The leaves of bergamot (*M. didyma*) may have the same effect, as both contain an oil that acts as a germ-killer, fighting fungi and bacteria.

Boil 250 ml of fresh leaves in enough water to cover, for about 5 minutes. Cool slightly, then apply wet leaves to irritated skin for about 10 minutes.

planting Sow seeds in full sun to shade, and in loose, rich, humusy soil.

cultivation Self-sows. Clip the flowers after they fade to control, if desired, or smother any errant seedlings with mulch.

harvest Cut foliage any time for use fresh or dried. Dig roots in autumn. Shake seedheads into trays for a week of further drying.

Myrrhis odorata
sweet cicely

Looking very much like a fern when not in bloom, sweet cicely forms a clump of feathery green leaves that stay fresh through most of winter. Also known as liquorice root, this perennial herb holds the sweet scent of anise in its leaves, stems and seeds, as well as its fleshy, fingerlike taproots. Rub a leaf and you will quickly smell the trademark aroma. (That sniff-test is also a

good way to check the plant's identity: both poisonous wild hemlock and harmless Queen Anne's lace can look similar to this herb.)

Two similar-looking plants share the name and attributes of sweet cicely. *M. odorata* is European and *Osmorhiza longistylis* American. Use the foliage, root or seeds to sweeten teas or flavour baked goods, soups, fish and potatoes.

salad in a saucer

A 7-cm-deep plastic plant saucer is ideal for watercress and saves on watering chores. Pour in 1 cm soil-less peat-based potting mix and fill with water. Poke in a few stems; they quickly grow aquatic roots and will produce foliage above the water.

Nasturtium officinale
watercress

The deep green leaves and crunchy stems of this aquatic perennial add a peppery bite to salads and are great in a chicken-stock potato soup. It is rich in vitamin C, iron and iodine, and before vitamin C was available year-round, watercress was eaten to treat scurvy. Its juice was used as an expectorant to clear the lungs, and was even rubbed on scalps in the hope of restoring hair.

planting Easiest to start by rooting a few fresh stems. Strip the lower leaves and insert stems in loose, moist soil. Keep soil well watered during growing season. A spot near to a pool or tap is ideal.

cultivation Mulch to keep moist and clean. Cabbage butterflies may lay eggs on them.

harvest Cut stems of leaves before they form flower buds, when the flavour turns bitter. Use fresh.

Nepeta cataria
catnip

If Kitty is your best friend, you'll definitely want to plant this herb to send her into fits of delight. Your planting may look a little battered after it endures the rubbing and rolling of feline ecstasy, but this hardy perennial herb will quickly spring back, ready for another round. Interestingly, some cats seem entirely unmoved by catnip. Instead of acting intoxicated, they ignore the plant. Researchers theorize that some cats are genetically unsusceptible to nepetalactone, the chemical in catnip and related hybrid catmint (*Nepeta* x *faassenii*) that triggers the reaction.

Catnip is a bushy, self-sowing perennial that can quickly turn weedy. If you want to make a big brood of catnip mice for gifts, its vigorous nature is a good trait. Grow it in a raised bed or cottage garden, where it can self-sow at will.

For a more controlled garden, try catmint (see photo, right), which does not self-sow. Besides being more compact, it yields hazy billows of blue-purple flowers that look great with roses, iris, poppies and other perennials.

planting Start with young plants or ask a friend for a few cuttings; they root in about a week. Grow in sun to shade, in almost any soil.
cultivation Allow space around the plant so that feline friends have easy access.
harvest Clip entire plant at base before flowering to dry for crafts or minty tea. Cut catmint flowers soon after they open for fresh bouquets or drying.

Ocimum spp.
basil

Your first armload of homegrown basil will make you feel like a blue-ribbon gardener. Basil is heady stuff – highly aromatic, super prolific, and as simple to grow as marigolds. For a small investment in a packet of basil seeds, you can harvest about a year's supply of this first-rate culinary herb. Bring on the tomatoes, the mozzarella, the chicken, the pasta, the prawns: with basil in your garden, your cooking is about to take an inspired leap.

Sweet basil (*Ocimum basilicum*) is the name for the traditionally scented annual herb. It has a strong, sharp aroma with a heavy hint of liquorice and a spicy warmth – a unique flavour that most folks enjoy from their first bite. Slice the leaves onto a frozen pizza, whirr them into pesto, simmer them in sauces. Almost any Italian dish tastes better with a little basil. Because the flavour is so dominating, however, use basil with a light touch until you know the preferences of your friends' and family's palate.

The popularity of plain old basil has inspired plenty of 'new and improved' versions with fancy leaves or unusual scents, plus a host of rediscovered exotic basils, including Thai, African and clove-scented varieties. Sampling the many types of basil available is a fun way to expand your sensibilities, but be sure to leave enough room for the regular all-purpose variety alongside the curly basil, the cinnamon basil, the lemon basil and the miniature basil. The extra-large leaves of 'Lettuce Leaf' basil will save you time de-stemming when you're ready to mix up a batch of pesto.

Grow basils in large pots or containers and place outside mid-June to early September, while the nights are relatively warm. It is best to make a group of pots in a sunny, sheltered area. The most reliable and best volume of leaves will, however, be obtained by growing in an unheated greenhouse or conservatory.

planting All basils are easy and fast to grow from seed, although multipacks of plants are also available. Plant in well-drained, average to fertile soil, in full sun.

cultivation Clip back every two to three weeks to encourage new leafy growth and delay flowering. Learn to recognize seedlings of this annual.

harvest Cut leafy stems or pick individual leaves anytime; the flavour is best before the flowers open. For large quantities, cut the entire plant at ground level. In cold areas, cut basil at ground level when frost threatens.

quick, easy pesto and variations

Basic Mix 500 ml fresh basil leaves, 3 cloves garlic, 30 g pine nuts and 250 ml olive oil in a blender. Process until a thick paste. Toss with hot pasta, spread on toast, dab on pizza or use as a dressing for sandwiches. Freeze any extra in an ice cube tray, then unmould them and put in zip-top freezer bags.

Cheesy Add 125 g Parmesan and 60 g Romano or Asiago cheese to the basic recipe. Great on muffins with tomato, breaded aubergine as well as poached scallops.

Walnut Substitute walnuts for pine nuts in basic recipe. Tasty with cheese-filled ravioli or Hungarian pierogies

(potato dumplings). Or split a loaf of French bread, dab with pesto and chèvre cheese, and grill until toasted and the cheese is melted.

Lemon Add juice of 1 large or 2 small lemons to basic recipe. Great with fish or chicken dishes or serve with hard-boiled eggs and grilled chicken salad for an easy brunch.

Oenothera biennis
evening primrose

This tall biennial is a 'must' in a herb garden or a herbaceous border. It is one of the most noteworthy herbs, with modern scientific research backing many of its claims; it is also a charming easy-care flower for meadows and cottage gardens. The flowers will actually open while you watch, with an almost audible snap and release of light, sweet perfume – this magical show takes place around sunset from mid- to late summer. Oil extracted from its seeds has been used with great success to alleviate symptoms of premenstrual tension and trials have seen many eczema sufferers experience improvement. The oil may also alleviate hangovers, depression, arthritis, obesity and acne, and is being studied for treatment of multiple sclerosis. The wonder-working substance is gamma-linolenic acid (GLA), also found in borage seed. Stay tuned for further developments in research and future products introduced to the public.

planting Easy from seed. Forms a rosette of leaves the first year and blooms the next. Plant in sun to part shade, in well-drained, lean to fertile soil.

cultivation Self-sows moderately. Flowers open late evening and close by mid-morning. Look for visiting moths soon after the flowers open.

harvest Not recommended for home medicinal use. Enjoy it in the garden with purple coneflower, asters and other summer-into-autumn flowers.

Origanum majorana
sweet marjoram

Sweet marjoram is lighter in flavour than its delicate cousin, spicy oregano. Beware of mislabelled plants; confusion reigns among the oregano clan. Although sweet marjoram is frost-tender, it grows rapidly and forms a large, sprawling mound in a single season. The flowers attract butterflies and other nectar-seeking insects, among them a multitude of wasps and other beneficial insects that will help control pests in other parts of your garden.

Grow sweet marjoram along rock walls, where it can spill among the stones, or let it trespass onto pathways, where its lively scent will be released by the occasional tread of passers-by.

Use sweet marjoram as you would oregano: in Italian cooking, with beef or chicken, in soups and sauces or on grilled vegetables. Mash a few leaves with butter and use for corn on the cob or baked potatoes. It also adds a piquant note to potpourri and sachets, without smelling like you accidentally sprinkled on the pizza topping.

planting Buy young plants from a reputable source; sniff before you buy if possible. Plant in light, very well-drained soil of poor to average fertility. Also thrives in large containers.

cultivation Start new plants from seed in early spring. Harden-off before planting out in mid-May. Half-hardy, protect if there are late frosts.

harvest Cut leafy stems any time. Collect large amounts before they bloom, for use fresh or dried.

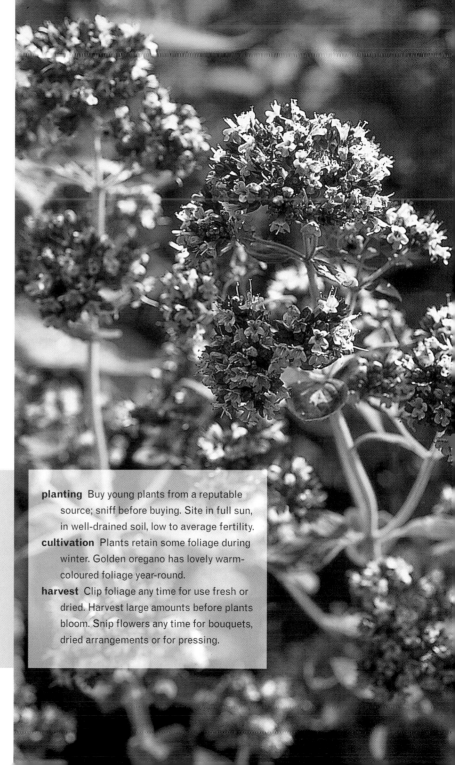

Origanum vulgare
Greek oregano

The pungent biting flavour called 'oregano' has its origin in plants found in the Mediterranean area. There are many variations in this plant's height and flower colour. Plant specialists offer the mild forms of origanum as 'marjoram' and the pungent flavoured one as 'oregano'.

The further south you travel in the British Isles, the more likely you are to see this pretty plant in wild areas or along clifftops. The rosy pink flowers attract butterflies and insects, but the leaves are mild.

Do keep a big patch of oregano in your herb garden, because you'll want plenty to use fresh and dried. The pungent, spicy flavour is a key note in tomato sauces, pizza toppings, Italian beef stews and many other dishes. Try it with grilled vegetables, potatoes, in scrambled eggs or bean dip, or mixed into cream cheese for use on bread or crackers.

take the sniff-test before buying

Oregano plants vary widely in their smell and flavour – some with barely any scent at all and others strong enough to make your mouth water for spaghetti. Seed-grown plants are usually insipid; look for plants grown from cuttings or divisions of strong-smelling parents. Always sniff before you buy. Even young plants will release the strong, characteristic odour of oregano when you bruise a leaf.

planting Buy young plants from a reputable source; sniff before buying. Site in full sun, in well-drained soil, low to average fertility.

cultivation Plants retain some foliage during winter. Golden oregano has lovely warm-coloured foliage year-round.

harvest Clip foliage any time for use fresh or dried. Harvest large amounts before plants bloom. Snip flowers any time for bouquets, dried arrangements or for pressing.

plant for the future

Ginseng is a long-term investment, not in money but in time. The roots take at least 7 years to develop to usable size and older is even better. As the desired root chemicals are diluted by fast growth, it won't help to douse it with fertilizer.

Pick a shady, undisturbed site – under sugar maples is its chosen habitat in the wild – and plant a small patch for the future. Prepare soil by digging in large amounts of chopped leaves composted until they crumble into loose, black soil-like material: the same stuff you find in the forests where ginseng grows. Plant young roots (or seeds), and do not disturb for a decade. Let autumn leaves lie in place.

Panax quinquefolius
ginseng

Once a common wild flower of Asia and North America, ginseng today is rarely encountered in the wild. Greed is the reason for the plant's decline. Its healing roots were sought not only by countryfolk, but later by speculators who combed the forests and sold the plants at extremely high prices for export to the Chinese market. Ginseng grows very slowly, needing about seven years to grow marketable roots, so unscrupulous collectors soon dug themselves right out of a job.

The long, fleshy ginseng root – often shaped like a crude human figure – is the powerful part of the plant. Esteemed as an aphrodisiac and all-around health enhancer, ginseng is held to be as vital to mental acuity as to physical well-being.

Grow ginseng in a shady garden, amongst ferns and wild flowers, such as may apple, wild blue phlox and bloodroot. In autumn, its shiny red berries add a flash of colour; pluck off a ripe berry and you'll see that it is shaped like a plump, puffed heart.

planting Buy young plants from a nursery, or sow seed in early spring in a heated greenhouse. Plant in moist, humusy soil, in the shade.
cultivation Mulch with chopped leaves to keep the soil moist. Do not cultivate nearby to avoid disturbing the root.
harvest Should your ginseng crop mature to the point you can spare a plant, dig roots in late autumn.

Papaver spp.
poppies

Beautiful, ruffled poppies are renowned for the stress-reducing effects of some species – most notably, the opium poppy (*P. somniferum*), a lovely annual with grey-green leaves and blooms in hues of pink, red and purple. Naturally, you won't be growing them for nefarious purposes, but you can indulge a passion for poppies by growing any of the perennial or annual types.

The red poppies of Flanders fields (*P. rhoeas*) immortalized in fund-raising paper flowers sold by veterans, are simple to grow from seed. Both field and opium poppies (available in narcotic-reduced strains) produce copious amounts of tiny black seeds, which make a tasty topping for muffins and other baked goodies, although they may show up on sensitive drug tests.

Plant poppies in a large patch to enjoy a sweep of silken-petalled colour. Or scatter seed in a cottage garden or informal flowerbed, where they can mingle happily with columbines, daisies, irises and other early-blooming summer flowers to great effect.

planting Sow seed for annuals directly in garden; seedlings are nearly impossible to transplant. Grow in full sun, in well-drained, fertile soil.
cultivation Annuals self-sow. For lasting poppies, try perennial Orientals; propagate by root cuttings.
harvest Pick almost-open buds for display; sear stem ends. Use seed capsules in dried arrangements. Shake ripe seeds into paper bag for culinary use.

Pelargonium spp.
scented geraniums, pelargoniums

You can make an entire herb garden from just scented geraniums. Dozens of cultivars with mouth-watering aromas and a delicious variety of form and foliage make it an exercise in self-restraint to limit yourself to just two or three. Luckily, it's easy to fit these agreeable tender perennials into the garden: they stay in tidy, branching clumps, so you can use them as accents, plant them as edgings or grow them in windowboxes or containers to showcase a single specimen or display a whole range.

Start your collection with the classic rose geranium, whose lobed leaves lend a pleasing flowery scent to cakes and teas. Add the extra-curly foliage of lemon geranium, a smaller plant with a neat, upright habit. Make room, too, for apple geranium, a relaxed plant, perfect at the edge of a large pot, where its soft gray, rounded leaves and delicate, white flowers can spill over the rim. Then fill in any gaps with your favourite scents: chocolate, geranium, nutmeg, orange, coconut, peppermint, eucalyptus and just about any other aroma you can think of. All are great for flavouring desserts and drinks and scenting cosmetics; the leaves themselves are not eaten.

Unlike traditional red windowbox geraniums, the flowers of scented geraniums take a backseat to the foliage. There is an incredible variety of leaf shape and size, from round leaves the size of a thumbnail to bold, lobed leaves almost as big as your hand. Many display beautiful variegation, with crisp white margins or snow-speckled foliage. Chocolate peppermint offers wide, green leaves splashed with brownish purple. Several types sport velvety grey leaves, with and without creamy trim. Oakleaf, which has a unique spicy scent, bears leaves that are shaped like that of a white oak. Flowers are usually pink or white, and tend to have a delicate, airy look.

apple geranium afterbath soother

1 Bruise 6 to 10 apple geranium leaves. Stir into 250 ml extra-light olive oil, in a small pan.

2 Set on low or warm heat, stirring frequently to release oil from the leaves into the mixture.

3 When oil is fragrant and very warm to the touch, remove pan from heat, cover and cool. Strain and funnel into a bottle with a squeeze top. After a shower or bath, smooth the oil sparingly on skin.

planting Buy young plants; scented geraniums are started from cuttings. Plant in full sun to part shade, in well-drained fertile soil.

cultivation Pinch off tips to encourage more compact growth. Start cuttings in midsummer for plants to winter indoors. Take spring cuttings for planting outside, when all frost has passed.

harvest Clip individual leaves or sprigs any time. Cut flowers for pressing soon after opening.

Perilla frutescens
perilla

Ruffly, aromatic perilla is an Asian herb that often turns up on plates of Chinese, Korean and Japanese food. Also known as shiso, it can be eaten in all stages of growth. When sprouting, it garnishes food with spicy red or green colour. The leaves are gathered in large amounts for cooking as veg or for use like seaweed in sushi and tempura. The spikes of small, fresh flowers are also delectable and the seeds can flavour plum pickles and other sweet-and-sour foods.

The red-leaved form of perilla is now favoured as a garden plant. Along with old-fashioned balsam and spiderflower, this undemanding annual passed from one gardener to another in town and country gardens and can now be found providing deep patterns of colour in many gardens, keeping company with venerable peonies and antique roses. Its strong colour contrasts well with almost anything.

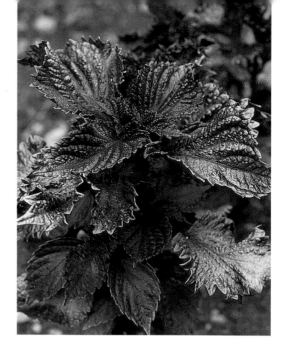

Perilla today is enjoying a renaissance, both for its decorative appeal and its tasty culinary possibilities. It also attracted attention recently due to the discovery that the oil from its seeds contains omega-3 essential fatty acids, famous for their potential to lower cholesterol. Once thought to be primarily a product of fish oils, omega-3's are now known to also be contained in some plant seeds, including flax and perilla.

The various forms of perilla available include those with plain or ruffled leaves of either red or green colouring. The red form mixes particularly well with petunias, zinnias and other annuals, where it may self-sow each year. Let it mingle with bearded iris, perennial geraniums and coreopsis. It can also be a useful and pretty addition to a shade garden.

planting Easy from seed, sown directly in the garden in full sun to part shade, in well-drained soil.

cultivation Drought tolerant, shade tolerant. Pinch off the tips to keep plants bushy and compact, or let them grow to their full height of about 60 cm. Seed spikes, which look something like those of mints, add a touch of delicacy to the winter garden.

harvest Best used fresh. Cut back plant halfway to harvest large amounts of the foliage. Cut the flowers any time for fresh use. Shake seeds into a paper bag when ripe.

Petroselinum crispum
parsley

Too bad so many sprigs of parsley go uneaten on restaurant plates – that little garnish of greenery packs a powerful punch of vitamin C, iron and the natural antiseptic, chlorophyll. Besides its healthful effects, a nibble of parsley has a solid practical use for those dining out or in: it will erase any lingering hint of garlic or fish on the breath. Old-time herbalists believed that eating parsley warded off the intoxicating effects of overimbibing in wine, perhaps an attribute to swallow with the proverbial grain of salt.

In cooking, parsley is valued for its ability to notch up the flavours of other foods. It is a staple in Italian recipes and adds a richer flavour to beef stew, poultry stuffing and vegetable casseroles. Its own flavour quickly lessens in cooking, however, so if you're making something less assertive than a tomato sauce, add parsley near the end to keep its distinctive savoury sweet taste. Chopped leaves liven up rice, grilled vegetables and fish, and are delicious in mild cheese spreads. Try parsley butter, made with fresh, frozen or dried leaves, on new potatoes, crusty bread or corn on the cob.

Plain or curly is the question when it comes to parsley. Both are similar nutritionally, but flat-leafed 'Italian' parsley is often more pungent, and the springy, tightly ruffled leaves of curly are used chiefly as a garnish. Grow within reach in pots, along walkways, as a ferny accent or as a rich green edging to a bright flowerbed.

planting Seeds can take months to germinate. Sow a row in spring for next season's use, but buy young plants if you want a guaranteed crop within a matter of weeks. Grow in full sun to part shade, in rich, well-drained soil.

cultivation Parsley is biennial: it forms only leaves its first year, then flowers and dies the next. Plant anew each year for a continual supply.

harvest Pick leaves any time. Use them fresh or freeze them. You can also dry parsley, although it tends to lose a lot of its flavour this way. For large quantities, cut up to half the leaves from the plant just above soil level.

easy freezing

Keep a supply of fresh-tasting parsley on hand by freezing it in zip-top plastic bags. Loosely stuff each bag with whole leaves and lay flat until frozen. Crumble the bag in your hand to 'chop' frozen parsley before use.

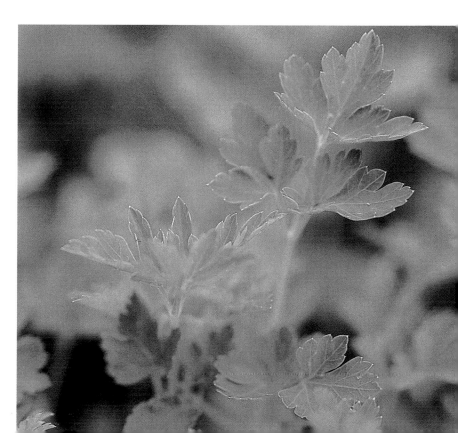

Pimpinella anisum
anise

Liquorice isn't only for the sweet counter. Its warm cloying flavour is tasty in grown-up treats, too, including baked goods, fruit soups, Indian cuisine – and of course adult-only liqueurs and aperitifs. Before you fire up the still to make a batch of homegrown Pernod or anisette, however, try the delicious liquorice flavour of this annual herb in something that the whole family can enjoy: a comforting cup of warm tea or a batch of savoury biscuits.

Fragrant anise has the alleged ability to stimulate the tastebuds into wanting more, which is probably why you can't eat just one black jellybean. Although its use has been largely out of favour for a number of years, anise has been enjoying a renaissance as ethnic recipes are revived and shared. For an unusual summer treat, crush some anise seeds with a rolling pin and mix them among ice-cold watermelon chunks.

planting Easy from seed. Sow in a sunny spot with well-drained soil.

cultivation Self-sows. Grow in its own bed or allow seedlings to crop up serendipitously. Looks like a spindly Queen Anne's lace.

harvest Gather foliage any time for use fresh, dried or frozen. Shake seedheads into a paper bag; let seeds dry for a week before storing in jars.

Potentilla spp.
potentilla, cinquefoil

Anything that could halt a toothache was treasured in the days before preventive dentistry and potentilla root quickly became a staple in the home herb supply. More than 400 species answer to the name *Potentilla* and herbalists tended to concentrate on a few favourites that are close at hand. While Europeans were packing their painful teeth with the root of their local species, for example, natives of Mexico and the American desert were chewing on a plant native to their area. Various potentillas were also used for dysentery, jaundice, gonorrhoea – and for tanning leather, a tribute to the potency of the astringent root. The cheerful red leather trim of Laplanders' reindeer-fur outfits was dyed with the root. You're likely to come across a member of this tribe as a weed in your garden; or you may choose to invite in any of the cultivated species for their abundant blossoms, which look like small wild roses.

planting Grow from purchased plants for bloom the same year. Plant in sun, in well-drained soil.

cultivation Highly adaptable and long-lived. Choose a permanent site; the taprooted plant is difficult to transplant.

harvest Do not use medicinally. Press flowers and interesting foliage of weedy or cultivated species for notecards and crafts.

Prunella vulgaris
self-heal

This useful plant often shows up in the rogues' gallery pictured on bottles of weed-killer, next to dandelions, violets and other plants that dare to infiltrate precious lawngrass. Before you reach for the spray bottle, consider all the good this unassuming little creeper once did. Made into a tea, it banished worms and stopped internal bleeding. Sore throats or tonsillitis were soothed after a good gargle with it. Smashed and applied to fresh wounds, it halted bleeding and speeded up healing. It was even used to expel devils from the afflicted, putting an end to supernatural fits.

Give self-heal a small patch for its creeping stems to spread and root into a thick mat. In late spring, and sporadically through to late autumn, it is decorated with short upright spikes of deep blue-purple flowers that are beloved by bees and butterflies. The plants also make a good ground cover; mix them with daisies and Roman chamomile for a small herbal lawn.

planting Easy to grow from plants transplanted from the lawn or purchase young plants. Grow in full sun to light shade, in average soil.

cultivation Propagate by division at any time during the growing season; stems root quickly. Thrives in wet soils as well as those that are well drained.

harvest Collect fresh leaves in summer and brew into a tea for gargling or to soothe burns or cuts.

Pulmonaria officinalis
lungwort

'Wort' shows up a lot in plant names, because it means exactly that: 'a plant'. In this case, the wort has leaves shaped like a human lung, round at one end, pointy at the other, and frequently spotted. Ancient herbalists practising the Doctrine of Signatures, in which plants were selected according to the body part they resembled, took one look at this perennial herb and used it on those patients whose wheezing breath or hacking cough indicated that perhaps their lungs resembled lungwort's blotchy leaves.

Interestingly, they weren't too far wrong, although their reasoning may have been a little sketchy. Lungwort is an effective expectorant, perhaps because its leaves contain silica, an irritant to the respiratory system.

If you want to experiment, stick to brewing a mild tea and using it very occasionally. But feast your eyes on lungwort all you like – it really stands out in the shady garden. You'll find a whole parade of lovely cultivars, with leaves stippled, marbled, spotted and blotched with white and cream. The pink or blue flowers are a sign of spring and are just as fleeting, but the foliage remains glorious all season, lighting the garden with dappled silver. Combine the simple shape of lungwort leaves with plain-coloured hostas or ferns. It spreads moderately in moist, humusy ground, forming a significant clump. The leaves dry nicely to add an unusual touch to potpourri or to pressed-plant crafts.

planting Buy young plants; lungwort self seeds, but all fancy cultivars are divisions of the parent plant. Grow in part to full shade, in moist but well-drained soil that is rich with humus.

cultivation Water regularly and mulch with chopped leaves to keep soil moist and loose. Propagate by division after flowering. Prone to drought-induced mildew; if leaves discolour, cut off affected leaves at ground level and allow to regrow.

harvest Collect leaves after flowering and dry them for tea or crafts.

Rhus glabra
smooth sumac

A few shrubs add permanent structure to a herb garden and they also remind us that not all herbs are soft green plants. Many woody plants were used medicinally, as early civilizations experimented with the possibilities of plants. Sumac, a group of American shrubs, was used by native Americans in doctoring a number of common ailments. Smooth sumac was one of the most widely used, although staghorn and shining sumacs were also of value.

Brewed into a tea, the sour lemony berries reduced fever and soothed sore throats and mouth sores. Roots and branches were made into a decoction to treat gonorrhoea, a trick that was quickly adopted by the European colonists, who were likewise troubled with the affliction. Boiling the leaves and berries made a mash that relieved the infuriating itch of poison ivy and mosquito bites, which were a real plague on the outdoor societies of the time.

reduce smoking by sipping tea

One native American use of this small tree may show promise to modern civilization: smooth sumac was used to lessen the desire for smoking tobacco. Apparently the strong addictive quality of nicotine was a problem even then.

To try it yourself, steep 1 teaspoon of ripe smooth sumac berries in 250 ml boiling water for about 20 minutes. Add a little honey to counteract the sourness of the fruit. Swallow a mouthful of the brew whenever you get the urge for a cigarette.

If the tea doesn't satisfy the cravings, you can also try smoking its dried leaves: they were used as a substitute when real tobacco was not available.

'officinalis': it's official

As you leaf through catalogues and references, you'll see some plants include the word 'officinalis' in their name (for example, *Pulmonaria officinalis*, *Salvia officinalis*). That's a clue that the plant was once held in high esteem by herbalists. Keep in mind, however, that the word is no guarantee of efficacy: it only indicates the plant was sold as a herb and widely accepted as a herbal treatment.

planting Buy young plants; they are tricky to identify in the wild and some (with white berries) are highly toxic. Plant in sun, in well-drained average soil.

cultivation Spreads by roots into a colony of small, suckering trees. Cut off shoots, or let it colonize a meadow or sunny bank, where its red autumn foliage and berries will be assets. Cutting down the parent will induce a spate of progeny.

harvest Cut foliage any time in season. Cut berries after a few frosts. Detach clusters to dry for teas.

Rosa spp.
roses

You would think that any plant that can cure the bite of a mad dog, regrow the hair on your balding head and 'make a face look young' would be tops in the garden – and thus it is with roses. Of course, the enduring popularity of roses has more to do with the beauty of the flowers than the unfounded claims of herbalists of yore. They are simply irresistible, with their lavish blooms, soft or saturated colours and that unmistakable fragrance that thankfully is being restored to modern hybrids.

Roses look great nestled amongst perennials or annuals, where their height adds variety to the bed. Plant lavender, thymes, artemisias, salvias and other low growers around their feet to blend bushes into the garden. Be sure to keep them within sniffing distance, though – a big part of the pleasure is inhaling their heavenly scent.

Rugosa roses and many old shrub roses, plus a plethora of modern hybrids, are nearly carefree. Unfortunately, that can't be said for dozens of others. As the rose craze swelled, less attention was given to survival than to making the biggest, boldest, best-looking flowers. Nowadays, though, you will find many of these flowers bred specifically for their hearty constitutions. Read the fine print on labels and in catalogues to find out if the rose you've fallen in love with is disease-resistant.

Planting a mixture of types will give you roses from spring through until frost. In mild climates, they bloom right the way through winter. One of the delights of growing roses is that unexpected last flower of the season, which usually shows up long after the peak of the show, as days grow shorter in autumn. The last rose of summer is more a thrill than all the abundance of June.

The fruit or 'hips' have been treasured herbally for thousands of years. High in vitamin C, the hard red or orange berries were packed for long sea journeys, and later collected by volunteers to keep British soldiers healthy during World War II. Brew a cup of rosehip tea yourself as preventive medicine against winter colds and flu. The petals also pack a punch: their astringent properties tighten the skin and shrink pores. The edible petals add colour strewn atop iced cakes or fruit salads.

rose follies and fancies

Beloved roses figure in myths and fairy tales, the classics of Shakespeare, war, religion and of course romance. If the price of a Valentine's Day dozen makes you shudder, consider Cleopatra: the sails of her ship were soaked in rose water so that perfume announced her arrival. The Roman Emperor Heliogabalus literally smothered his guests by filling the room with so many rose petals there wasn't much space to breathe. At the other extreme Saint Francis of Assisi supposedly turned his mind from temptation by rolling in a thicket of thorny rose canes whenever a lowly urge threatened his serenity.

planting Plant bareroot roses in early spring; plant potted roses any time. Choose a spot in the sun, in rich, loose, well-drained soil.

cultivation Monitor for black spot, aphid infestations, rust and other problems; remove affected parts. Rake up fallen leaves to minimize pests and diseases. In very early spring, prune and thin roses, removing dead canes and cutting back dead branch tips to a healthy bud. Hardiness varies.

harvest Cut flowers for bouquets. Collect petals for culinary or craft. Gather hips when they change colour late autumn; dry in arrangements.

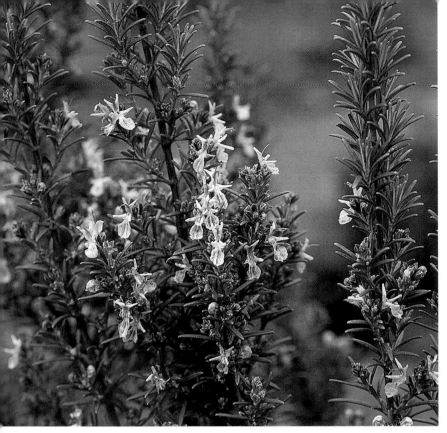

Rosmarinus officinalis
rosemary

With its stiff, skinny leaves and piney fragrance, rosemary could be mistaken for a downsized conifer. But what a mistake that would be. This aromatic shrub imparts delicious flavour to lots of our favourite dishes, from spaghetti sauce to grilled chicken to oven-roasted potatoes. Long-lived in milder climates, rosemary becomes a permanent player in the garden, thriving for decades. Many cultivars are available, from low-growing prostrate forms that look beautiful spilling over a stone wall to 2-metre-tall, bushy types ideal for hedges. You can indulge in it wherever you live: It flourishes in containers and grows to good size in just a single season.

Very popular in cooking, rosemary infuses mild foods with its flavour, making magic with grilled fish, baked aubergine and tender lamb. Both dried and fresh leaves are highly aromatic. Add it to casseroles, soups and tomato sauces, toss in salad and pasta, lay leafy stems on baking chicken, fish or meats and use to flavour oils and vinegars, or to scent cosmetics and bath oil. To shoo mosquitoes, rub a fresh sprig on bare skin.

Abundant spikes of small, pale to dark blue, pink or white flowers in spring and summer, and year-round deep green foliage make rosemary valuable in perennial beds, too. Plant taller cultivars to frame your doorway, or flank a bench with plants within arm's reach. For a summer pot, combine it with sulphur-yellow 'Moonbeam' coreopsis and a ruff of white petunias.

planting Seeds are slow to get started; buy young plants. Grow in light, very well-drained soil, full sun.

cultivation Susceptible to scale; snip off affected branches. If you see delicate webbing on the branches, spray upper- and undersides of foliage vigorously with water to dislodge spider mites. Do not allow soil of container plants to dry out. In cold areas, mulch plants with a deep, light layer of dead leaves for winter protection. Propagate by layering or take cuttings of young branches in summer.

harvest Snip foliage any time for use fresh or dried.

Ruta graveolens
rue

The softly textured blue-green foliage of rue is too good to ignore, but handle this herb with care: many people find they are allergic to the foliage, which can cause a blistering rash. Even seedlings pack a wallop. To prevent mishaps, keep it in flowerbeds, where its lacy leaves, mounding form and unusual colour make a fine partner for other perennials.

It was popular for its metaphysical properties, among them warding off witches, devils and evil spells, as well as enhancing 'second sight', the ability to predict the future. More prosaically, it was used to heal tired eyes and headaches. Forget about employing this herb for healing: not only is the foliage too risky to handle, its bitter alkaloids can cause spasms and even death.

Rue may irritate the skin, but it is decidedly delicious to the eye. For a romantic summer garden, nestle its soft foliage around a patch of pale pink, old-fashioned shrub roses – and add a collar of honey-scented sweet alyssum to keep the rue out of reach.

planting Sow seed in pots or buy young plants; always handle with gloves and long sleeves. Grow in full sun, in well-drained, lean to fertile soil.

cultivation Wearing protective clothing, prune back in early spring to encourage dense, compact growth; otherwise, the plant may become loose and sprawly. Drought tolerant; this herb adds lushness to a dry garden.

harvest Ornamental use only. Do not touch with skin.

Salix alba
white willow

Pussy willows are a favoured sign of spring, but these trees and shrubs once had many more uses. Their thin branches were woven into mats and baskets; the bark was collected in spring to ease fever, pain, infections and upset stomach.

Willows usually grow beside streams where their roots can suck up the water they crave. Invite them into your garden with care: the roots will seek out reliable sources of water, including underground pipes.

planting Plant a young tree in sun to part shade, at least 30 metres away from any underground pipes. Or grow in a wooden half-barrel.

cultivation Willows grow very fast, which creates weak wood that is prone to breakage. Prune back hard in late winter to keep in bounds.

harvest Saw off branches and strip bark in spring; soak 1 tbsp of bark in cold water for several hours, then boil for 10 minutes. Swallow the bitter decoction one mouthful at a time until the pain subsides – or pop an aspirin instead.

the first aspirin

Nibble a branch of white willow and you'll taste a familiar bitterness: salicin, the forerunner of today's ubiquitous aspirin, infuses the bark of this tree. For more than 2000 years, folks reached for willow bark instead of the aspirin bottle.

Salvia officinalis
culinary sage

If you only know sage as dusty leaves in a jar on the spice rack, get ready for a pleasant surprise. Fresh sage has an unusual but lovely camphor-bitter lemon scent, a big improvement over the musky smell of the dried leaves. Sample this strong-flavoured herb in small doses at first. Chop some fresh leaves to strew across omelettes or drop into canned or fresh tomato soup, or bruise a few leaves and simmer in a cream sauce to serve over pumpkin-stuffed ravioli. Enjoy sage in its traditional role in poultry stuffing, pork roasts or sausages, and experiment with the herb in lentil, rice and nut dishes, in mushroom or barley soups and with grilled, baked or steamed onions, potatoes, marrow, carrots, aubergine and other veggies.

While we think of sage as a herb to simmer in sauces and stir into stuffing, the ancients slugged it down straight, as a steaming tea. Sweetened with a dab of honey, sage tea is a soothing drink that will reduce symptoms of a cold, as well as laryngitis and a sore throat.

planting Easy from seed or buy young plants. Grow in well-drained, average to fertile soil, in full sun.
cultivation Cut back young branches in late winter to keep vigorous and compact. Couple the grey foliage and rich blue flowers with bright, silky poppies, daylilies or roses. Good in containers, too. Propagate by cuttings or layering.
harvest Pick leaves any time for use fresh or dried.

Salvia spp.
sages, salvias

So many salvias, so little garden space – culinary sage has roughly 750 relatives in the large genus whose Latin name translates roughly to 'salvation'.

One of the most dramatic is pineapple sage (*S. elegans*), a shrub-size beauty that explodes in autumn with bright red flowers at the tip of every branch. Its foliage smells sublime, so plant it where you can catch a whiff in passing and be sure to dry some for potpourri. Clary sage (*S. sclarea*) is an old-fashioned cottage garden plant, another big one that tops out at about 1 metre tall and wide. Its unusual flowers get added colour from bracts that may be tinted pink, purple or blue. Try its leaves instead of culinary sage in recipes.

Three ornamental salvias stand out: the hybrid *Salvia* x *sylvestris*, with its neat mounded habit and abundant deep blue-purple blooms, which bless the garden from late spring through autumn; fire-engine-red scarlet sage (*S. splendens*), planted as a bedding annual since the turn of the last century; and blue salvia, or mealy-cup sage (*S. farinacea*, especially 'Victoria'), grown as an annual.

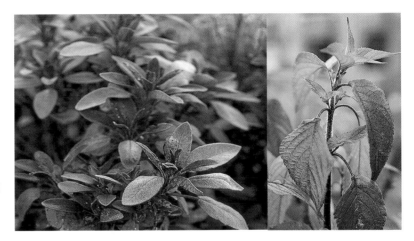

colour in autumn

The tubular, nectar-rich blossoms of salvias – especially the red variety – are highly appealing to insects, and the spikes of outward-facing flowers are perfectly arranged to fit their hovering habits. During late summer and autumn the many herbaceous salvias come into bloom, including the blue or white *Salvia patens*, the beautiful purple *S. gesneriiflora* as well as many others. The pretty coloured bracts of annual *S. horminum* are a particular favourite of flower arrangers.

planting Grow from seed started early indoors for flowering the same year, or buy young plants. Grow in well-drained, average to fertile soil, usually in full sun.

cultivation Choose salvias according to where you intend to use them in the garden; heights, habits and bloom times vary widely. Easy to propagate by cuttings. Hardiness depends on species.

harvest Nip off individual flowers soon after they open to dry for potpourri or crafts. Pick leaves of aromatic cultivars anytime for potpourri or cooking.

Sambucus spp.
elder

During the Middle Ages, folks spent a lot of time trying to keep away evil spirits, which apparently must have been raising quite a ruckus. Elder was one weapon in this battle: plant it by the door and no bogeyman could enter; neither would the house be struck by lightning, nor assailed by witches. Of course, figuring out the habits of evil spirits was no easy job: contrasting lore held that elder was actually the home of witches, which disguised themselves as branches.

Country people also made a tea from its roots to induce labour, relieve headaches and clear mucus from the lungs, and simmered the flowers to wash sore eyes. Elder was prized for its berries, which make excellent wine and jam as well as a decent cough syrup. Dipped in batter and then fried, the wide, flat blossom clusters – picked clean of insects – make tasty fritters topped with a dusting of icing sugar. Dried and used in cosmetics, the white flowers have a reputation for bleaching freckles and whitening the skin.

Children of old also used elder, whittling the hollow stems into whistles or pipes, a hobby that may have caused nasty side effects. The stems, roots and leaves contain cyanide-like elements and have a strong laxative effect. Skip the medicinal uses, but do gather berries to make jam and wine. Be sure to strain out all seeds, which contain toxins. And imbibe sparingly, as the fruit has a bowel-loosening effect.

planting Buy young plants. Common elder (*S. nigra*) has dark purple fruit; *S. racemosa*, red berries; *S. caerulea*, blue berries. Grow in well-drained soil, in sun to shade depending on species.

cultivation Elders grow fast and spread quickly by underground roots. Give them a patch of their own, with a fence upon which they can lean their berry-laden branches. Hardiness varies depending on the particular species.

harvest Clip blossoms soon after opening. Swish in water to rinse out insects. Pick berries when fully coloured. Songbirds adore the fruit.

Sanguisorba minor
burnet

Close your eyes and sniff – is that a cucumber you're smelling, or a sprig of burnet? This ferny, perennial herb is perfect for sparking up salads, especially in spring when real cucumbers are hard to come by in the garden. The delicate leaves of burnet must be used fresh from the garden, but you'll be able to gather them for most of the year, even in much of winter.

Burnet loses flavour with cooking, so add it to soups and sauces at the last minute. Blend finely chopped fresh leaves into cream cheese or butter to spread on crackers, fish or hot corn on the cob. You can use a stem of dainty leaves as a swizzle stick in mild mint teas or in ice water.

The taproot of a related perennial herb, great burnet (*S. officinalis*), was once used to tan leather and was occasionally employed medicinally although its high tannin content can affect the kidneys and liver.

Both species often escape from gardens and can be found growing wild in fields and roadsides in some areas of the country.

planting Easy from seed, or buy a young plant. Grow in full sun to light shade, in well-drained, lean to fertile soil.

cultivation The plant becomes lanky after flowering. Cut back to ground level and it will quickly put out new growth. Self-sows; clip faded flowers before they go to seed to reduce progeny.

harvest Cut leaves any time for fresh use or to press.

elder flower wrinkle cream

Lacy white elder flowers were prized for their skin-tightening effects. Why not test their alleged abilities yourself? Dry blossom heads, face down, on a clean net curtain. Crumble a generous handful into a bowl, and gradually mix in a few tablespoons of plain yogurt until a thick paste is formed. Slather onto wrinkle-prone skin areas. Wait 15 minutes, then splash off with cold water and pat dry.

Santolina chamaecyparissus
santolina

Santolina is great to practise topiary skills on. With regular shearing, it grows dense and full and is easy to train into formal or fanciful shapes. This perennial shrub holds its leaves all year, which makes it a favourite for knot gardens, low hedges and decorative borders.

Both deep green and silver-leaved santolinas are available. Their year-round colour is equally valuable in the garden and dried arrangements. In midsummer, the plants are topped by a crowd of neat yellow or cream button flowers, which can be dried to add colour to arrangements.

Take advantage of the softening effect of this herb by planting it along pathways or patios. Grow it in containers or windowboxes, too; its delicacy complements large-leaved scented geraniums. You can also use the quiet colour of silver-grey santolina to calm a flower garden of hot colours, or as a step between clashing hues, such as not-quite-complementary roses.

planting Sow the slow-growing seeds in pots, or buy young plants. Grow in full sun, in well-drained soil of poor to average fertility. Rich soil causes lax plants and poor foliage colour.

cultivation Cut back hard in early spring to make it bushy. Repeat after flowering, removing the flower stems and branch tips. Propagate by cuttings or layering in spring, or divide large plants.

harvest Clip foliage in spring and summer, cutting whole stems. For drying, snip flowers with long stems soon after they open.

goodbye moths

Santolina looks light and delicate, but it carries a heavy-duty scent that will make your nose wrinkle with its unexpected pungency. That super-strong aroma makes santolina an effective anti-moth treatment. Dry and crumble the foliage into a square of cotton, knot the ends and hang in a cupboard or drawer amongst jumpers or silks.

Saponaria officinalis
soapwort

A froth of pink flowers that completely cover the spreading plants is soapwort's greeting to the warm days of summer. In its homelands of Europe and Asia, it covers large expanses with sweeps of colour, and in North America, where the herb has escaped from gardens, it blankets roadsides with a solid swathe of pale pink that continues sporadically through the first frosts.

Like many old favourite flowers, soapwort comes with a list of nicknames: bouncing Bet, old maids' pink and dog cloves were some of its aliases. It was also called bruisewort, because of its reputation for healing skin problems. No nicknames were assigned to this easy-care perennial for its other uses, as an expectorant, a gout treatment and a last-ditch effort against the growth of tumours. The root of soapwort is where the medicinal properties are concentrated. A decoction made from one heaped tablespoon of dried root in a cup of water was swallowed one mouthful at a time for an all-purpose dosage for targeted ailments.

Soapwort is most famous for the sudsy wash water made from its roots and stems, which contain saponin. Farmers used it to clean sheep before shearing, while cloth-makers washed their homespuns in it. Don't expect a high lather, as the dirt-cutting power of this natural soap relies on chemical action more than bubbles.

Give it plenty of elbow room in the garden. Its leaves are covered with a greyish bloom, like grapeskins, so even when not in flower it makes attractive ground cover, especially interspersed with rocks. Shoulder it with Siberian iris and other upright perennials for contrasting form or let it meander among the cosmos and bergamot of a cottage garden. The pink, sometimes white, flowers have a light, sweet scent.

planting Seed is slow to sprout and must be planted in autumn. For faster results, take cuttings from the wild in summer, or buy young plants. Grow in sun, in well-drained soil. Fertile soil leads to invasive growth; lean or stony ground slows the spread.

cultivation Pull up the creeping roots when they overstep allotted boundaries. Propagate by division or cuttings. May self-sow.

harvest Collect stems any time. Cut stems of flowers soon after opening for fresh bouquets. Dig roots in autumn and dry for later use.

lather up: camping trip shampoo

Travel-size plastic bottles make home-made shampoo more of a fun experiment than a necessity on modern camping trips, but it's still nice to know that the means to clean your hair exists in the wild, just in case the Millennium bug shows up later than we thought. Gather two generous fistfuls of soapwort stems, clip them at ground level and chop them coarsely. Combine with about 250 ml water in a pan or a bowl and stir them vigorously to release the saponin. Strain and use as shampoo or laundry soap. This recipe is still used for old curtains and tapestries.

Satureja hortensis
summer savory

Just as its name suggests, this annual herb makes foods taste better. Its peppery flavour has hints of thyme. Often overlooked as a possibility for the cook's garden, savory turns ordinary side dishes like peas, green beans, baked or boiled potatoes, marrow, cabbage and lentils into treats that will make friends and family lick their lips and ask for more. Use its lively flavour to wake up fish, beef and chicken recipes, too. To add a spicy tang to fried chicken or other breaded foods, mince fresh savory or crumble dried leaves into the bread crumbs. Summer savory tea eases stomach cramps and diarrhoea. It also has a long-standing reputation as an aphrodisiac, perhaps because of the way its sprightly flavour awakens the senses.

planting Easy from seed sown in sunny, well-drained soil of average to rich fertility.
cultivation As foolproof to grow as marigolds, summer savory requires attention only when its seedlings are very young, to prevent them being overshadowed by competing weeds.
harvest Gather foliage any time for use fresh or dried; flavour best before bloom. Clip to delay bloom and keep vigorous; once it sets seed, growth slows.

Satureja montana
winter savory

This is a perennial relative of summer savory, with a stronger personality and a coarse, piney flavour that needs an assertive companion food. Use it with venison and other game, or in patés. You can also mince it into breadcrumbs for preparing trout or other fish or chicken.

Curiously, one medicinal effect of winter savory was supposedly just the opposite of its summer cousin: instead of enlivening the libido, it was believed to quell sexual desire.

The fine leaves of this nearly evergreen perennial make it ideal to weave into knot gardens or train as a low hedge. It likes frequent shearings, growing bushy and dense. Its rich, deep colour is held through all but the hardest winters, maintaining a garden's structure as well as providing fresh flavour year round.

planting Hard to grow from the fine, erratic seed, so best to buy young plants. Grow in full sun, in light, very well-drained soil of average to rich fertility.
cultivation Add gravel or sand and compost to lighten heavy clay soils, or grow in free-draining pots.
harvest Clip foliage any time. Use fresh or dried in cooking. For an unusual fresh wintertime bouquet, combine glossy sprigs with a bit of holly or dress up its vase with a red bow.

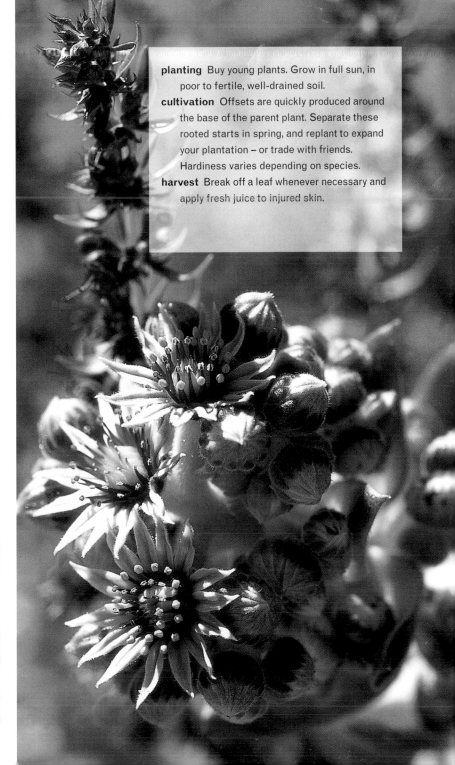

Sempervivum spp.
houseleek, hens-and-chicks

Houseleeks are best known as ornamentals or rock plants, but they once held a secure foothold in herbal lore. These pretty, succulent rosettes, available in an array of shapes, sizes and tints, are almost as soothing as aloe when broken leaves are applied to burns or slight cuts. You can also use the juicy leaves to take pain out of insect bites, sunburn and even irritation caused by herbs such as nettles or rue. *S. tectorum*, one of the largest houseleeks is also the one most used for first aid.

Most of the cobwebbed or more colourful types are usually found in the alpine section of garden centres and nurseries. These tough plants thrive in places no other plant can grow. They snuggle happily into the merest crack in paving or rock walls. For a little surprise, fill a pedestal birdbath with potting soil and add a few starts. In the herb garden, they add lively texture to fine-leaved creeping thyme.

success in a strawberry pot

Tall containers with pocket planting holes around their sides are called 'strawberry pots', although it's very difficult to grow juicy berries in them. Due to the arrangement of the pockets, soil at the roots of plants dries out rapidly. Instead of struggling with strawberries, fill these pots with houseleeks, which thrive even in drought conditions. Push the roots of each plant firmly into place in the pocket, and settle a few at the top of the container. They will quickly become established and begin producing little offsets that hug the sides of the pot.

planting Buy young plants. Grow in full sun, in poor to fertile, well-drained soil.

cultivation Offsets are quickly produced around the base of the parent plant. Separate these rooted starts in spring, and replant to expand your plantation – or trade with friends. Hardiness varies depending on species.

harvest Break off a leaf whenever necessary and apply fresh juice to injured skin.

Serenoa repens
saw palmetto

This palm-like shrubby plant once covered vast areas in the southern states of America, but today colonizes only a fragment of its original holdings, despite the sprays of berries becoming a hot property in the market for nonprescription herbal preparations.

Traditional herbal use esteemed the dark purple or black berries as a source of healing teas, particularly effective on respiratory ailments like bronchitis and asthma. Congestion is also said to be alleviated by sipping a cup or two of saw palmetto berry tea each day. If you suspect serious health problems, get the advice of a medical doctor before trying herbal remedies that may not be as effective as traditional modern medicines.

Saw palmetto is one of the hardiest of palms, but still needs a subtropical climate in order to truly flourish. You can try to cultivate it as a houseplant or summer patio plant if humidity levels are high. Daily sprays with a fine misting device, to replicate the summer showers in its native habitat, also encourage its growth.

If you decide to test this herb's hardiness outside, it is prudent to grow it in a container for some years because fully mature, established plants are also decidedly more tolerant of cold. Be sure to give it winter protection and only plant it in a permanent garden position when its sheer size dictates. When this time comes, transplant it into a warm corner, well sheltered from the wind, and give it plenty of water.

As you will discover, saw palmetto has a unique growth habit, with the thick, almost trunk-like root remaining below the ground and only the tuft of bold leaves waving above the soil.

planting Buy a potted plant. Transplant, when ready, in part to full shade, in sandy, fast-draining soil.

cultivation Clip off dead leaves as needed with secateurs. May be successful in a large container filled with lightweight soil-less potting mix. Supply a little supplemental moisture by misting the foliage daily in dry spells. Once established, will tolerate temperatures down to 5–10°C.

harvest Berries ripen in mid-autumn through winter. Clip the bunches, strip off the berries and spread on screens to dry.

health benefits

Saw palmetto tea is supposed to increase sexual powers, a claim which may have led to one of its more modern uses. Today's herbalists have turned to the plant as an aid for prostate problems, an advertisement now under closer scrutiny by science. Early investigation shows promising results, and over-the-counter users are snatching up the hoped-for cure. The burgeoning number of asthma sufferers, too, are sampling saw palmetto, which has a long-standing reputation for soothing breathing difficulties. Because over-the-counter herbal preparations are mostly unregulated by the government, experimentation with this alternative treatment is a personal decision.

Solidago odora
goldenrod

A territorial thug, goldenrod is notorious for swallowing up more than its share of the garden. Its fast-spreading roots crowd out anything in its path. Yet sweet goldenrod (*S. odora*) and others of its ilk were once valued cures for everything from bee stings to flatulence to kidney stones.

Include goldenrod in a meadow garden, or grow it with bergamot, autumn asters and other tenacious types. Roots are fairly easy to get rid of, and self-sown seedlings can be hoed off or hand-pulled. The sprays of golden flowers are unsurpassed for attracting beneficial insects and butterflies on autumn migration.

planting Seed is hard to find; start with young plants. Grow in full sun, in well-drained, lean to average fertility soil. Rich soil encourages faster spread.
cultivation Pull unwanted roots.
harvest Cut flowers soon after opening for fresh or dried bouquets, or to mash into a lotion for insect stings. Collect fresh anise-scented leaves any time to steep as a medicinal tea.

not the hay fever culprit

Goldenrod comes into full bloom just as hay fever sufferers are reaching their sneezing, itchy-eyed peak. The real culprit is usually tree or grass pollen, or even the ox-eye daisy, which blooms along our hedgerows. Unlike goldenrod, their pollen is windborne, so it easily reaches unfortunate noses.

Stachys officinalis
betony

One of the most widely used medicinal herbs, betony was good for curing dozens of complaints, or at least so proclaimed old-time herbalists. Science is still working to prove or disprove the claims. It is known to contain tannins, which are bitter substances that act as astringents, drawing out moisture. Old herbals recommend it for bronchitis, sore throat, profuse sweating, vein problems and worms, an affliction thankfully rare these days. A simple use for the juicy stems is to apply them to minor cuts or skin blemishes. An old name, lousewort, refers to the odd belief that it caused sheep to become infested with lice if they ate it.

A cousin of betony, the velvety grey lamb's-ears, is better known by gardeners than this green-leaved perennial. The spikes of reddish purple flowers attract bees and other nectar lovers, and will even bring butterflies. Betony is a tall herb, with spikes as tall as a metre. You may encounter it in shady, wild places where it has leaped out of an old garden. Purple coneflower and goldenrod make good partners.

planting Easy from seed. Grow more ornamental named cultivars from young plants. Plant in full sun to shade, in well-drained soil of average fertility.
cultivation Some varieties tend to spread; uproot as required. Propagate by division.
harvest Collect leaves any time for making tea. Press individual flowers for paper and other crafts.

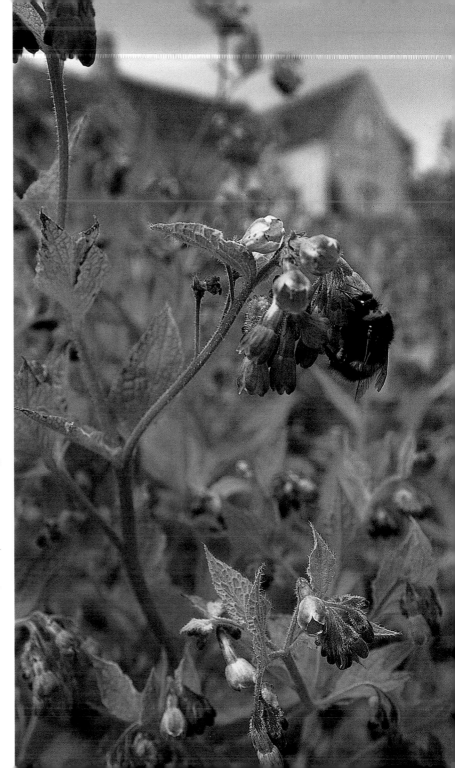

Symphytum officinale
comfrey

Stout and coarse, comfrey is an emphatic plant that's impossible to overlook. Its handsome leaves can reach almost 30 cm in length, and the plant in bloom towers to 1.5 metres. Comfrey blooms are fascinating to watch unfurl from buds. The flowering stem emerges in a tight coil of pink-tinged buds, and slowly relaxes into a curved stem strung with dangling blue bells.

It has been implicated as a liver carcinogen, so avoid comfrey internally. But do savour the knowledge that this stout herb once alleviated stomach, menstrual and gastrointestinal distress. Externally, it is safe to use and speeds healing of cuts and burns. Boil the leaves and fish them out to make a poultice for minor wounds, insect stings and other skin problems.

Once you plant comfrey, it's there to stay, so choose a site with care before you invite this deep-rooted perennial in. Removing adult plants is tedious because new growth sprouts from bits of broken roots. Add the slimy rhizomes that gave the plant the nickname 'slippery root', and you have another reason to keep it undisturbed.

planting Sow seed or buy a young plant; one is all you need unless you're planning a comfrey hedge. Grow in sun, in well-drained soil of lean–average fertility.
cultivation Cut back hard if it topples, or support with sticks. Pull out self-sown seedlings.
harvest Collect fresh leaves any time. Press individual flowers for crafts.

Tanacetum balsamita
costmary

Fans of micro breweries and home brewing should get to know this lesser known herb, which was once wildly popular. Formerly known as alecost, this sturdy perennial was prized by brewmasters, who added its spicy, slightly minty leaves and flowers to all their beer. Meanwhile, on puritan church pews, costmary was known as Bible leaf, thanks to the custom of tucking a sprig among the pages of the Good Book, both to mark the place and to impart an occasional whiff of sharp fragrance to clear a drowsy head after a long sermon.

Aromatic costmary is just as delightful in a steaming bathtub after a long day at work. You can also slice slivers of fresh leaf among boiled potatoes or into soups, salads and poultry stuffing for a savoury tang. Use it sparingly until you decide how strong you like its bold flavour.

planting Seed is difficult; start with young plants. Grow in sun, in fertile, well-drained soil.

cultivation Costmary flowers look like they belong on a different plant: they are sprays of small, delicate white daisies held atop the 1-metre-plant. Clip off flowers after they're done blooming.

harvest Pick fresh leaves any time. Cut flowers for fresh bouquets. Dry leaves and flowers for potpourri or sachets.

Tanacetum parthenium
feverfew

A dainty cousin to costmary, this perennial puts forth a flurry of small white daisies above its airy, bright green foliage. Its common name is a matter of some dispute; apparently the plant was used more to dispel headaches than to alleviate fevers. Research is ongoing as to the herbalists' claims that feverfew cures migraine headaches; studies have turned up interesting side effects, including improved sleep and less arthritis pain. Whether these are wishful thinking or due to ingesting feverfew remains to be seen. Treatment, in any case, is less than pleasant owing to the bitter taste of the leaves.

Feverfew is a generous self-sower, but its offspring are always welcome. Young plants are easy to transplant to other locations, and their long bloom period – from rose season in early summer to michaelmas daisies time in autumn – makes them a garden treasure. The masses of tiny white flowers mingle easily with lavender, catmint, salvias and other flowering herbs.

planting Easy from seed; plants sprout in as little as 5 days. Grow in full sun to part shade, in well-drained, average to fertile soil.

cultivation Self-sows or propagate by division. Often short-lived, but self-sowing ensures a new batch of feverfew every year.

harvest Pick leaves or sprigs of foliage to dry for use in pest-repellent sachets.

Tanacetum vulgare
tansy

Tansy is one of the most commonly grown herbs, probably because it's also one of the easiest to grow – and therein also lies the problem. A particularly enthusiastic self-sower and a fast spreader, tansy quickly forms stout clumps of roots so thick that you can barely get a spade into the clump. Unfortunately, except for dried flowers, tansy is also one of the least useful herbs. Its pungent foliage was once used in embalming and to expel worms, two applications that the modern herb gardener generally has little use for. Made into sachets or laid in among your clothes, the foliage can make a decent insect repellent.

planting Easy from seed or buy young plants for bloom the same year. Grow in sun to part shade, in well-drained soil.

cultivation Keep tansy in a meadow or cottage garden, where its pushy ways won't become a nuisance, or confine to a large container to keep in bounds. Clip off flowers before they set seed to minimize self-sowing.

harvest Clip flowers for drying soon after they open. Gather the foliage any time to dry for use as an insect repellent.

second round of flowers

Feverfew blooms most abundantly in summer, then continues to push out new clusters of its small white daisies for sporadic bloom through frost. To get a second full burst of fresh flowers, cut back the plants by about one-third after blooming. They will quickly produce new branches, reinvigorating the plant, and form a host of new buds.

Taraxacum officinale
dandelion

Ever wonder how all those yellow flowers ended up dotting your lawn? Thank the efficient seed dispersal system of the widely despised dandelion, which sends its myriad seeds airborne, each equipped with its own mini-parachute, all set to make a landing and plague lawn lovers everywhere, raising up their proud yellow heads as soon as the sun begins to shine in the springtime.

Dandelions are now so widespread throughout the world that their actual point of origin is somewhat in doubt: most authorities are content to settle on Eurasia, but of course this still encompasses quite a lot of ground.

Although lawn care companies have been supported for decades by the anti-dandelion crowd, there is a multitude of reasons to appreciate instead of annihilate this plant. First of all, it's downright tasty. Young leaves have a refreshing, slightly bitter flavour that perks up salads and soups. Tight flower buds contribute the same flavour with a satisfying bite-size crunch, although older buds are undesirable because their petals tickle the throat. For a sunny touch on casseroles, salads and soups, tear apart a blossom and scatter some yellow petals across the surface. If you want to try a new zing in your coffee or cocoa, chop the dried roots into 5-cm pieces, roast at 150°C for about 10 minutes, grind and add about a quarter teaspoon when brewing a cup.

Dandelion gets its name from the French *dent de lion*, or lion's tooth, referring to the jagged leaves. Amaze your children by making dandelion magic: slice the bottom part of a flower stem into strips, using your fingernail. Dunk in a glass of ice water and the strips will instantly curl into tight coils.

planting Sow a row of the large-leafed variety with your vegetables to make harvesting easier than scouring the lawn. Plant in sunny, well-drained soil; if you intend to harvest roots, dig in liberal amounts of compost so that soil is loose in texture.

cultivation Invest in an inexpensive dandelion digger tool to evict self-sown strays.

harvest Pick leaves when young for mildest flavour. Older leaves are good in soups. Pick flower buds when small to medium size and tightly packed. Dig roots in autumn for drying.

spring tonic or winter delight

To herbalists, dandelions are a dream come true. The plant is used by countryfolk as a spring tonic for its actions in stimulating the liver and kidneys to remove toxins from the body. Exactly how this occurs is explained by an old name for the plant: 'piss-a-bed'. High in vitamin A, vitamin C and potassium, the tangy leaves invigorate a tired body after a winter with no fresh greens. Tea made from the leaves has been used to cure constipation and upset stomachs; a stronger infusion from boiled roots allegedly helps gallstones. To remove troublesome warts or corns, rub the milky juice from leaves or stem onto the skin. If all else fails, try a nip of dandelion wine, a legendary beverage to make you forget what ails you.

Thymus spp.
thymes

Variety is a big part of the fun with thymes: these tiny-leaved perennial herbs come in all sorts of colours, textures and personalities. There's culinary thyme, for instance, which grows into an upright, bushy mini-shrub infused with that familiar scent. Woolly thyme, a love-at-first-sight herb, crawls closely along the ground, making a blanket of fuzzy foliage that begs to be touched. Lemon thyme bears green leaves and a clear sharp citrus scent. Add variegated types with white-edged foliage (see photos, far right); those with flowers in pink, red, purple or white (see right); those that smell like nutmeg, camphor or caraway – you can fill a whole garden with thymes without ever getting bored.

Thyme is easy to use in cooking, too, because its flavour marries well with just about anything. It makes all kinds of meats, poultry, fish, game, stews and soups taste better. On the vegetarian side, it peps up rice, lentils, beans, potatoes and

quick chicken dinner

1 Cook enough rice or pasta for four servings.

2 Cut two chicken breasts into small chunks. Heat 2–3 tbsp olive oil in a frying pan,

add chicken and sauté until meat is opaque.

3 Drain a jar of roasted red peppers and add to pan, with 2 cloves garlic, minced, and 2 tsp fresh

thyme, chopped. Stir until chicken is tender, about 10 to 15 minutes.

4 Add chicken medley to rice or pasta. Garnish with sprigs of thyme.

other starches, and adds zip to any vegetable – from artichokes to courgettes. Mash it into butter for bread or corn on the cob, simmer it with garlic and rosemary in marinara sauces, make flavourful vinegar – the list is endless.

Aromatic thyme is also delightful in the bath, in lotions, in potpourri and sachets. It improves digestion, soothes a cough, eases asthmatic breathing, helps headaches, encourages sleep and relieves flatulence. You can tuck it into herbal wreaths and dried arrangements.

Create a sampler in a large container, fill windowboxes, tuck creepers among cracks in paving, cover sunny slopes, make a thyme lawn or combine with flowers. The fine texture makes a luscious underpinning for roses – and will also release a lovely fragrance when stepped upon.

planting A few thyme species are easy from seed sown in pots, where you won't have to spend time weeding among the tiny seedlings. For most of the good culinary or beautiful varieties, buy young plants or beg a start from a friend. Plant in full sun, in well-drained soil of poor to rich fertility.

cultivation Drought tolerant. Propagate by cuttings or division. Protect marginally hardy types with a deep mulch of loose leaves. Start cuttings in summer for potted plants to winter on a windowsill.

harvest Snip foliage any time for fresh use or drying. To harvest large quantities, cut back plants by halfway in early summer; they'll quickly regrow.

Tropaeolum majus
nasturtium

Nasturtium flowers look like delicate exotics, but at heart they're homely, kin to the wild yellow mustards that blanket spring fields and the lowly shepherd's purse that finds a home at roadside. All are members of the giant mustard family. Nibble a leaf – or a flower if you can spare one – and note the familiar peppery bite of a mustard. Use its leaves in salads, its spicy flowers to dress up open-face sandwiches or add a confetti touch to salads and rice, and try the crunchy buds fresh or pickled like capers.

Gratifyingly easy to grow, nasturtiums have seeds the size of green peas, ideal for a child to handle. They sprout seemingly overnight, and bloom in just a matter of weeks. Grow trailing varieties in windowboxes indoors or out, and use the bright red, orange or yellow flowers to edge beds or add a dab of colour in pots. Insects adore the blossoms.

planting Easy from seed. Soak overnight in water for faster germination. Plant in full sun, in well-drained, average to fertile soil.

cultivation Although usually grown as an annual, nasturtium is perennial in very mild climates. Cabbage butterfly caterpillars may eat the leaves; plant more in another location and enjoy the butterflies that hatch. Aphids can sometimes prove troublesome.

harvest Pick leaves or flowers any time for fresh use. Grow indoors for winter salads.

Urtica dioica
stinging nettle

Take that name seriously. An up-close-and-personal encounter with this plant will leave your skin itching and burning for hours or even days. Stinging nettle has one of the most devilish arsenals in the plant kingdom. Beneath its leaves and covering its stems are zillions of tiny, hollow hairs that work like hair-trigger hypodermic needles. They actually inject their 'venom' into the skin of anyone unlucky enough to blunder into the plant – or even lightly brush against it.

All the same, stinging nettle has been popular for centuries – as food, medicine and for making cloth. One of the more bizarre uses to which the plant was put was described by the Roman, Petronius, who suggested that a cure for a lack of virility was to thrash the poor fellow with nettles in the, uh, nether regions. Less dramatic uses were achieved through nettle tea, said to relieve asthma and other breathing difficulties, diarrhoea, and urinary problems. Hopeful folks rubbed nettle-root brew on heads to stimulate new hair. Practise positive thinking and try a home-made hair rinse; it may not grow a fresh crop, but will give remaining locks a lovely shine.

In spring, these wild greens make nutritious cooked vegetables when picked young. (If the leaves are mature, the stinging hairs can cause internal irritation.) They are rich in vitamin C and mild in flavour. Prepare as you would spinach – but be sure to wear gloves and long sleeves when working with the greens.

Keep nettles in an out-of-the-way part of the garden and think twice about growing them if you have small children. Many butterflies seek out nettles to lay their eggs on; look for the caterpillars or evidence of nibbled leaves.

planting Grow from seed gathered in the wild, or beg a root from a friend. Plant in pots, where you can keep an eye on them and avoid accidental contact. Plant in sun to shade, in fertile, moist soil.

cultivation Wear protective clothing whenever you approach the patch. No care is needed; nettles will flourish just fine when left to their own devices.

harvest Gather young shoots as soon as they appear in spring, and pick young leaves for cooked greens. Snip mature leaves any time for hair conditioner. Always handle with extreme caution.

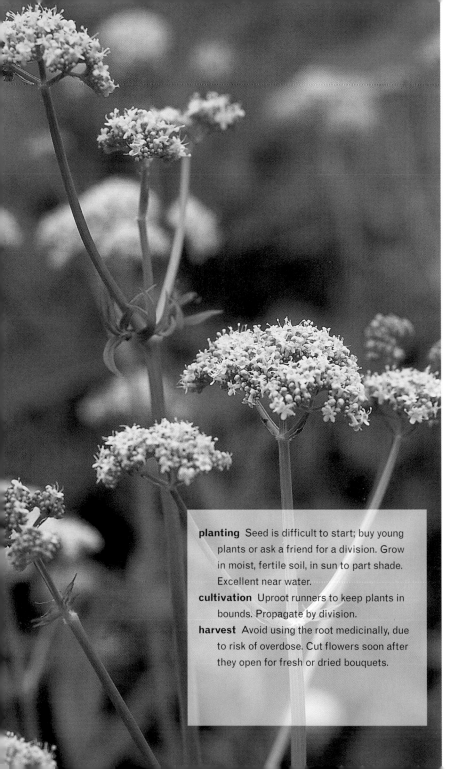

planting Seed is difficult to start; buy young
plants or ask a friend for a division. Grow
in moist, fertile soil, in sun to part shade.
Excellent near water.

cultivation Uproot runners to keep plants in
bounds. Propagate by division.

harvest Avoid using the root medicinally, due
to risk of overdose. Cut flowers soon after
they open for fresh or dried bouquets.

Valeriana officinalis
valerian

You are getting sleeeepy, very sleeeepy. If you
had just sipped a cup of valerian tea, it would be
no surprise to find your eyelids growing heavy:
the perennial herb has been used as a
tranquillizer for centuries. Scientists still aren't
sure just how valerian slows a body down, but
they do know that ingesting too much can lead
to dizziness, depression and eventually stupor.

Cats will find this herb equally intoxicating,
although they get that languorous feeling from
scent alone. They adopt a planting as quickly as
catnip, rolling in the foliage. Human noses have
a hard time understanding the lure, because
valerian can smell like stale sweat or old leather.

Growing to as much as 1.5 m, valerian spreads
into large clumps by underground roots and may
also self-sow. Although it isn't as widespread a
weed as other herbs such as chicory and
comfrey, valerian is often found growing in the
wild around old railway banks, as a stray in
meadows or along streams.

Valerian is also called garden heliotrope,
because at their best, the early summer flowers
have a sublime scent. The fragrance can vary
widely from one plant to another, so if possible,
take a test sniff of the flowers before you buy.
Dry the flowers for potpourri if you like the
smell. Plant it in the back of the garden, where
its clusters of tiny white or pinkish red flowers
will provide a soft backdrop behind bearded iris,
phlox and other summer-blooming perennials.

Verbascum thapsus
mullein

'Velvet plant' is one of over 30 common names for this biennial herb, which puts forth a rosette of big, irresistibly soft leaves its first year, then erects a woolly poker of yellow flowers in its second year, blooming intermittently from midsummer to early autumn. The tall, dark brown candelabra persist until spring, when they finally topple to make room for newcomers.

Mullein is a dramatic foliage plant for the herb or ornamental garden. The clump of soft, silvery leaves can spread to 60 cm across, making it as useful in the sunny garden as hosta is in the shade. The quiet colour works wonders with hot magenta petunias but also looks great with white flowers and silvery artemisias. Leave the stalk in winter to add height to the garden, and attract birds, searching out insects.

Brewed into a tea, the leaves stop wracking coughs and soothe irritated throats. The tea also calms digestive difficulties. To bring on sleep or quiet aches and pains, the flowers too can be

gathered for tea, using 1 teaspoon for each 250 ml of hot water. If you're suffering from congestion, make a tent over your head using a towel and breathe in the head-clearing vapours. Mullein flowers were also said to remove warts, and a poultice of boiled leaves may help heal cuts and abrasions.

worth a try as wart remover

Mullein's yellow flowers were just as valued by herbalists as the big grey-flannel leaves. To try them yourself as a home-made wart remover, crush a handful of fresh blossoms with the back of a spoon in a bowl. Pat onto the affected skin and wait about 15 minutes. Remove the flowers and allow the skin to dry. Reapply daily until warts hopefully disappear.

planting Scatter seed here and there in the garden in autumn or spring. Grow in full sun, in well-drained, lean to fertile soil.

cultivation Its deep taproot makes mullein difficult to transplant, so work around volunteer seedlings instead of trying to move them.

harvest Slice off leaves at their base with scissors for fresh or dried use. Collect the flowers soon after opening.

Verbena officinalis
vervain

Vervain's romantic story begins with the goddess Isis, shedding tears for her dead lover. Wherever a tear fell, so the story goes, vervain would then spring up.

Treasured since ancient times for its healing properties, vervain was believed to stop spasms, quiet raging fevers and heal kidney and liver afflictions. Applied externally, it was used for skin rashes and cuts. It was also sampled by men as a marital aid in pre-Viagra days.

Vervain tends to look more weedy than ornamental, but its skinny, branching spires of tiny, sparkling whitish flowers have an airy look that is pretty with bright red flowering geraniums or scented geraniums of interesting texture planted in front of it.

planting Easy from seed. Grow in full sun to part shade, in moist but well-drained fertile soil.

cultivation Pull out self-sown seedlings when young. Mulch to retain moisture.

harvest Collect leaves before flowering occurs in summer to autumn. Chop 1 tbsp and soak in cold water overnight to make a treatment for skin irritations. Avoid taking internally; nausea and vomiting can occur even with moderate doses.

Vinca major, V. minor
periwinkle

Well known as a reliable, free-blooming ornamental groundcover, periwinkle has a distinctive lavender-blue colour that is lovely with daffodils, tulips and other spring bulbs. Three species are commonly grown: *V. minor*, a popular evergreen ground cover; *V. major*, a taller and more vigorous type; and *V. major* 'Variegata' with bright green or gold leaves. All bloom early in spring and continue putting forth a few new flowers through much of the year.

Traditional uses included treating diarrhoea and haemorrhage: periwinkle's astringent properties apparently aid in stopping the free flow of various body fluids. Enjoy it for its beauty instead of its curative value: just gazing upon the sea of 'periwinkle blue' works wonders to calm you down. Both make dense, evergreen ground covers, beautiful with ferns or hostas for textural accent, or as a cloak for spring bulbs.

planting Buy multipacks of young plants in spring. Grow in sun to shade, in moist to well-drained soil.

cultivation Highly adaptable, growing well in a variety of soils and conditions. They spread fast through underground roots and may be invasive. Plant as ground covers. Propagate by division or cuttings.

harvest Do not use medicinally. Press the flowers for notecards and other crafts.

Viola spp.
violets, pansies

Old-fashioned charm is what you'll get when you plant violets. These carefree perennials are so easy to grow that they tend to be overlooked, despite their wonderful potential to add perfume and colour to cosmetics, drinks, sweets and syrups. Dozens of species of violets spread across the world, but by far the most commonly found species is the sweet violet (*V. odorata*), a hardy species with colour that lives up to its name. The world of violets rapidly becomes fascinating once you begin exploring: check specialist plant catalogues for burgundy-leaved Labrador violets, long-spurred dog violets, bright blue birdsfoot violets, downy yellow wood violets and dainty white violets.

One step away from violets are violas, which look more like small pansies than a nosegay of violets. Less cold-hardy, they're often planted in masses or in containers as early spring annuals. Pansies are ever popular, with romantic new colours and ruffled shapes showing up every year at garden centres. Recently, they've been bred specifically for improved cold tolerance, and winter pansies are now available in most garden centres during the autumn.

Once used medicinally, violets are today known best for their edible flowers. Dip small blossoms in sugar syrup for candied ornaments to top desserts, or use flowers to add colour to green salads, melon or fruit. Freeze smaller flowers in ice cubes to add pizzazz to ice water.

planting Some violet species can be grown from seed, but many are sold as young plants. Buy them in multipacks or start seed indoors in winter for spring bloom. In general, they prefer a shady or partly shady site with loose, humusy soil and plenty of moisture, but required conditions vary according to species. Pansies and violas thrive in containers.

cultivation Uproot strays or let them spread as a quaint ground cover. The rare pearl-bordered fritillary butterfly seeks violets to host their young.

harvest Pick blossoms soon after opening, for pressing or eating.

index

acknowledgements

My education as a herb gardener began at my mother's knee, searching out dandelions for a spring tonic and tying snippets of lavender into my father's handkerchiefs for sachets. I didn't realize what a thorough grounding I was getting in precious lore until decades later, when I would mention some such pastime to gardening friends, only to be met by blank stares. Didn't everybody know that chamomile worked better than expensive shampoos for making your hair gleam? Was I the only one that made my own teas instead of buying fancy boxed blends? For that early head start, I have to say, Thanks, Mum.

Gratitude goes to Jimmie Epler, too, who taught me the basics of botany over several seasons of outdoor jaunts, until I knew a mustard from a phlox without taking an exploratory nibble. Arch Judd taught me the importance of learning Latin, and gave me immersion lessons at his dinner table, where only botanical nomenclature was spoken. Lessons are everywhere, though, once you start asking questions, and I am also thankful for the many seasoned gardeners and practitioners who generously shared what they knew, whether by chance encounter in the woods or a long visit over the backyard fence. Lastly, Charlotte Beech, the editor of this book, is as rare a find as that elusive blue Himalayan poppy – her editorial eye and ear for language are as sharp as her sense of humour, which kept me laughing throughout. And that, as even herb gardeners will agree, is the best medicine.

picture credits

Page 10/11 Andrew Lawson RHS Chelsea 1999 Designer Terence Conran, **12** Derek St Romaine RHS Hampton Court 1999 Designed by Ruth Chivers, **16** Jules Selmes, **17** Glyn Barton, **21** Derek St Romaine RHS Chelsea 1998 Designed by Bunny Guiness, **24** David Murray, **26/27** Clive Nichols/Tonie Lewenhaupt Sweden, **28** (bot) David Murray, **35** Derek St Romaine RHS Chelsea 1994 Designed by Noula Hancock and Matthew Bell, **38** (left) Claire Nuridsany and Marie Perennou /SPL, **49** (top) Rex Butcher/GPL, **49** (mid) Howard Rice/GPL, **49** (bot) Lamontagne/GPL, **50** David Murray, **52** Derek St Romaine, **57**(right) Lamontagne/GPL, **86, 89** (top), & **91** David Murray, **95** Derek St Romaine, **98/9** J S Sira/GPL, **100, 101,** & **106/7** David Murray, **108** Andrew Lawson, **114/5** Howard Rice/GPL, **118, 123** (top), **125,** & **129** David Murray, **141** John Glover/GPL, **146** David Murray, **152** Derek St Romaine, **163** David Murray, **172** William Gray/Oxford Scientific Films, **174** & **178** David Murray